HEART FAILURE: OUR LIFE JOURNEY

*The life journey of a group of
Heart Failure Warriors*

Thomas Trimble,
Jerome Boeck and
Christopher Gehrke

CONTENTS

Jeff S.   Gatlinburg, TN (#26)
Christina S.   Lakewood, CO (#27)
Sue J.   Wellston, OH (#28)
Carol C.   Lockwood, NY (#29)
Dixie C.   St. John, NB, Canada (#30)
Lisa W.   Ogden, UT (#31)
Gerald   Mastic Beach, NY (#32)
Jeffrey M.   Ord, NB (#33)
Name Withheld   Calverton, NY (#34)
Virginia B.   Minot, ND (#35)
Shirley C.   Panama City, FL (#36)
Jim B.   Winchester, VA (#37)
Megan   Denver, CO (#38)
Bob H.   London, Ontario, Canada (#39)
Allison S.   Platte, SD (#40)
Name Withheld   Brookfield, WI (#41)
Tea M.   Gastonia, NC (#42)
Debbie F.   Philadelphia, PA (#43)
Jocelyn V.   Gordonsville, VA (#44)
Sheila M.   Philadelphia, PA (#45)
Darlene B.   Florence, SC (#46)
Cindi L.   Hillsboro, MO (#47)
Cordelia M.   Victorville, CA (#48)
Name Withheld   Cherry Hill, NJ (#49)
Teresa P.   Mt. Holly, NC (#50)
Cathy S.   DeWitt, AR (#51)
Carole C.   Houston, TX (#52)
Paul S.   Fort Wayne, IN (#53)
Lisa J.   Mio, MI (#54)
Ellen   Fremont, CA (#55)
Mark W.   Wheeling, WV (#56)
Suzy H.   Spring, TX (#57)
Name Withheld   Asheville, NC (#58)
Roxie A.   Conklin, NY (#59)
Amie K.   Florence, AL (#60)
Jesse M.   Las Vegas, NV (#61)
Leslie   Clarksville, IN (#64)
Jack K.   Hutchinson, KS (#65)
Chris T.   Sullivan, MO (#66)
Name Withheld   Brighton, TN (#67)

Robert B.   Annan, Dumfries and Galloway, UK (#68)

Name Withheld   Kalamazoo, MI (#69)

Name Withheld   Sanford, NC (#70)

Ciara B.   Triangle, VA (#72)

Sandy P.   Oklahoma City, OK (#73)

Martin A.   Birmingham, West Midlands, England (#74)

Dianne G.   Langley, British Columbia, Canada (#75)

Marcie B.   Shalimar, FL (#76)

Janet L.   Brooklyn, NY (#77)

Daniel D.   Ravenswood, WV (#78)

Name Withheld   Enfield, United Kingdom (#79)

Keith S.   Kinghorn, Fife, Scotland (#80)

Joe N.   Orland Park, IL (#81)

Sara B.   Mt. Laurel, NJ (#82)

Isabelle D.   Kitchener, Ont., Canada (#83)

Patricia R.   Dentin, MD (#84)

Kara H.   Apple Valley, CA (#85)

Scott D.   Wooster, OH (#86)

Gloria W.   Scott City, MO (#87)

Maribel H.   Ocala, FL (#88)

David K.   Opelika, AL (#89)

Steve D.   Franklin, TX (#90)

Mandy   Folkestone, Kent, UK (#91)

Nancy N.   Addison, IL (#92)

Malcolm W. Swindon, Wiltshire, England (#93)

Kim Z.   Mason, OH (#94)

Angela D.   Topeka, KA (#95)

David B.   Wales, MA (#96)

Jill T.   Dunnellon, FL (#97)

Toni L.   Smyrna, TN (#98)

Kathy A.   Long Beach, CA (#99)

Michael W.   Cleburne, TX (#100)

Mark F.   Derby, KS (#102)

Teresa S.   Daviston, AL (#103)

Laurie L.   New Sharon, ME (#104)

Carrie   Little Egg Harbor, NJ (#105)

Annette F.   Storvreta, Uppsala, Sweden (#106)

Dion M.   Brisbane, Queensland, Australia (#107)

Christy   Los Alamos, NM (#108)

Clay L.   Reno, NV (#109)

DEDICATION

This book is dedicated to the Millions[1] of people in the world who are suffering in the battle against Congestive Heart Failure or CHF. Most of these people will be in this battle for the rest of their life. A battle that takes every bit of your strength and energy to try to keep on with your life journey. We hope this group effort can help them with that fight.

We also thank the people who have volunteered their stories to help provide a Group Body of Knowledge, to share and help all these other people.

I also want to thank people like my co-authors, Jerome, and Christopher who take a large portion of their time to run Facebook Congestive Heart Failure Support Groups, trying to help some of these warriors while being in the battle themselves.

We hope you enjoy reading the individual journey of all of these people.

Thanks, Thomas Trimble

---

[1] According to the Centers for Disease Control (CDC) in 2018 there are 5.7 Million people suffering from CHF in the United States.

INTRODUCTION

All of our lives are a journey. Some parts of it we control other parts are totally out of our control. This book is a sequel to my previous book called, "HEART FAILURE: A Life Journey". That book documented my personal 30-year journey with **Congestive Heart Failure** also known as CHF.

Jerome Boeck and Christopher Gehrke, the co-authors of this book, run Facebook Congestive Heart Failure support groups and suggested the direction for this book. This time we are telling the story with the help of a lot of other people, presenting information from their journey in their world of CHF. These people have all volunteered to explain the impact on their life from CHF and all are members of these two Facebook support groups.

This is an attempt to help everyone share their problems, results, and approaches to getting better or just surviving as long as possible with this killer CHF. Together we will form a group "Body of Knowledge" that many people can benefit from possibly even the medical profession.

We realize the advantage of what I might call, "group learning". By sharing our experiences, symptoms, treatments and what we have heard from our doctors, it forms a collective knowledge.

Sharing this information helps with education, reducing fear from the unknown, understanding what may happen and providing a guide which can be shared with caregivers and people we contact in life. It may even be shared with some doctors to help them all understand our lives and problems better.

Each member's section will deal with one person's individual journey, what they have learned, their feelings, fears, and hopes for the future. Their section will provide some identification (only First Name and Last Initial for security and their location) and their own description of the journey they are taking.

On behalf of Christopher, Jerome and myself, let me thank all these people for their voluntary contribution to our group Body of Knowledge and hope it benefits all.

Let's get started and meet this very special group of people and listen to their stories.

MEMBER RESPONSES

This section of the book chronicals many people's life story with CHF. These people provided their information to make this book warm and human. As I stated, my two co-authors Christopher Gehrke and Jerome Boeck both have CHF and run Facebook support groups for people diagnosed with CHF, along with their family and friends. We ran a survey in each of those groups asking for volunteers to share their story specifically for this book. The information here is taken <u>only</u> from that voluntary survey and no information has been taken from the discussion posts in those <u>private</u> groups. The number shown to the right of each person's title line is only a reference back to their survey entry for documentation purposes.

In the process of assembling this book, I have had to edit some of the member's responses for spelling and word choice to make them understandable to everyone. I have taken great care to respect and not change the meaning of the member's entries.

The three authors have significant CHF stories. Our stories will start us off in this section.

We hope you enjoy all the group's stories.

Thomas Trimble   Las Vegas, NV (Author)

"I, unfortunately, am very experienced with CHF. I have been a CHF patient battling this condition for over 30 years since age 38."

The main symptoms I experience are:

"Severe shortness of breath, wet cough, dizziness, pain, Edema, weight gain, fatigue, exercise intolerance, anxiety, depression, brain fog, short temper, OSA, VTAC, and some 'unidentified' chest pains."

CHF has impacted my quality of life in many ways:

"Well, I am not sure I actually have "Quality of Life". I get short of breath sitting at my computer, let alone walking. It is almost impossible to complete daily tasks no matter how much my head says I should, my body says NO. Luckily, I am retired on a pension and SS, because I sure could not work anymore. I can drive, but my loving wife has to do all the things like shopping for groceries. So where is the Quality?"

The medications I am taking are:

"Ace inhibitor, beta blocker, Digitalis, two diuretics, Warfarin, along with meds for diabetes, GERD and allergies."

I am experiencing Depression I describe like this:

"I am in almost constant pain from any of several issues. I cannot accomplish anything I wanted to do with the rest of my life. I have symptoms while sitting in my recliner, try to do much of anything and it gets way worse. People often say they have a little man on their shoulder who is telling them what to do. In my case, he pretty much says well what else can go wrong and what are you going to do to end it."

I feel there are several worst things about CHF is:

"Feeling useless, the brain fog, short temper and the total inability to do anything physical."

This is the story I wanted to share:

"The story of my life with CHF is so long and complex, I wrote a whole book on it (Trimble, 2018)[2]. My CHF world started after a damaging silent heart attack at age 38 killed 25% of my heart. Caused, at least partially, by my stupidity in my younger life. The heart attack damaged my left Ventricle. I found out after a while that it damaged the electrical function of my heart too. That gave me Ventricular Tachycardia or VTAC. That then led to needing an Implanted Cardioverter Defibrillator or ICD. They become a permanent part of your life and I am now on ICD #5. The damage to my heart has continued to make it weaker and weaker. Many doctors and patients treat the measure of your Ejection Fraction or EF[3] like

---

[2] Heart Failure: A Life Journey; Published by Amazon/Kindle 2018, e-Book ASIN: B07GTRHQ5S and Paperback ASIN: 1719901171.

[3] Ejection fraction (EF) is a measurement, expressed as a percentage, of how much blood the left ventricle pumps out with each contraction. An ejection fraction of 60 percent means that 60 percent of the total amount of blood in the left ventricle is pushed out with each heartbeat. From Heart.Org

it is the whole story of your level of CHF. Last time it was measured my EF was 33%, but that does not really say the way I feel. If I were to guess, I would say I feel like a non-functional person with an EF of 10% or less. I have been through the pit of Anemia to the point where the lack of Iron in my blood made the breathing even worse when I didn't think it could get any worse. Then it was pumped back up with Iron IVs, a lovely Root Beer colored liquid. I was discovered to have Obstructive Sleep Apnea or OSA. Now after two Sleep Studies and a lot of insurance talking, I use a CPAP every night with oxygen connected to it. In fact, I have oxygen connect to me 85% of the day. Since we live in Las Vegas, we are surrounded by casinos. I love slot machines so we go there often. It also gives me a place I can walk around in air conditioning. Early in the morning, the smoke is not bad. Now my idea of a walk is a burst about 20 yards long, then stop and rest both because of leg pain and shortness of breath and that is with my trusty portable oxygen on. Based on the NY Heart Association scale, I am entering Class IV-D. That is my opinion because I cannot get any doctor to tell me theirs. Don't get me started on doctors and communication. That scale is definitely something you do not want to be rated in the top class. So 'life' goes on. My condition gets worse at whatever rate it feels like. My wife always feels I am not getting worse, but that may a be some wishful thinking. She says it while she is handing me my oxygen? Well, it feels worse from in here. I try to do what I can. I go to doctors, take the meds, try (I said try) to eat right and lose some weight and get my amazing 20 minutes of exercise a couple times a week. Doctors always have a severe hang up with overweight people and make it sound like losing weight cures everything. So I have seriously started working at doing that and have lost the first twelve pounds. My condition is one of the ones that will never get better, because of the damage to my heart. I can not get a transplant due to other factors. So, I am stuck hoping some genius scientist gets Stem Cells working for the heart or who knows what else. **Maybe, I will be here to see it?**"

Jerome Boeck   *Seguin, TX (Co-Author)*

Jerome has been in our CHF world for 4 years. He is the owner of a Congestive Heart Failure Support Board on Facebook.

The main symptoms he experiences are explained as:

"Sudden weight gain, Edema, Memory Loss, Shortness of Breath, Frequent Urination and Depression."

CHF has impacted his quality of life described like this:

"Prior to my diagnosis in December 2014, I was like Superman. Then my diagnosis became kryptonite. I went from doing anything and everything to being almost totally dependent on others for help. After my triple bypass in December 2014, I had to live with family until I was able to recover and return back to work. It has taken me a while to realize that I have a quality of life but it is a very different quality of life. With CHF you learn to find value in what you have and your family and friends become essential to your continued quality of life."

Jerome is being treated with medications:

"Heart failure medication, diuretics, a blood thinner, electrolyte supplements, antidepressant, receptor blocker (low blood pressure), statin (cholesterol)."

He is experiencing Depression/ Anxiety described like this:

"After my heart attacks and diagnosis of CHF, I developed depression. I was focusing on the negative and couldn't see that I was needing help. My focus was off at work and in my life. Everyone around me said I was different. I wasn't the same happy go lucky guy anymore. I was more drawn into myself and it was as if people treated me differently. I was told over and over to get help and maybe take something to help me. I knew I wasn't crazy and that I did not want to tell a stranger my problems. Especially when that stranger was not going to truly understand my situation. I did not want for a person with no health issues to tell me how to handle my issues."

He says the worst thing about CHF is:

"Working in health care for 30 years helping others and not taking care of myself to the point that my heart issues which led to CHF would have possibly been prevented."

This is the story he wanted to share:

"It was Thanksgiving Week November 2014! One of my favorite times of the year and I knew I would be busier than usual. I was only working three days. I was planning on going to see my family for Thanksgiving and cooking for everyone! I had the menu planned and shopping was done. We would be gathering at my brother and sister-in-law's house in Boerne. Alfred and Tonya almost always host holiday events.
I decided to go to work early that Monday morning to knock out some work while it was quiet and the phones wouldn't be ringing off the hook. I got to the office around 6:30 am and was met by Morris, the office cat. After getting into the office, I turned on the computer and started working. As a case manager/supervisor with a caseload of 20 consumers with developmental disabilities, I always had plenty of work to do. And with

five house managers reporting directly to me, my cell phone was always busy with the employee, consumer, and family issues. After working about 30 minutes, I started to feel like I had a fever. My body started to sweat profusely. I felt achy as though I was getting the flu as it was going around the office. Given the time, I decided to walk to my car and turn the AC on high. I actually fell asleep in the car and awoke to the sound of the overnight truck pulling into the office about 7:45 am. I met the driver and then went back to work. Throughout the day I felt like my energy was being drained from my body. Walking maybe fifty feet to the copier, I got out of breath. I continue to work and by Wednesday, I wasn't sure I could handle Thanksgiving weekend. I pushed forward still thinking it was the flu.

To help with coverage at the group homes, I chose to take a consumer with me for the weekend. Brian had been around my family and they liked him. He and I had a great together having known him since 2009 when I started with the company. I also had to pick up Tonya's sister from her group home and take her to Boerne as well. I packed the car, left San Antonio and we headed to Boerne to start cooking. I was still very tired and felt hot. The Thanksgiving meal went off without a hitch and everyone enjoyed the food as always. The day after, we all headed out to go to a peddler's trade show. We walked around all day. I felt tired and short of breath but didn't say anything. Brian and I separated from the others and we took lots of breaks to stop so I could catch my breath. By the end of the weekend, I was tired but no longer felt hot. We headed home and I went back to work on Monday.

During the next three weeks, I continued to work putting in over 40 hours a week. Despite working in an office, I still had to visit group homes, day programs and go to meetings. I walked a lot at our office as the copier and fax machine was in the office next door. I had to go upstairs occasionally. I also dealt with crazy staff who didn't help my stress level. I was part of the on-call rotation at work carrying a pager for two-weeks at a time. That meant being the go-to supervisor for emergencies for all eleven group homes within the company. I was babysitting Brayden, my four-year-old great nephew, and Cassidy, my eight-year-old great niece one a week. April, their mom was a nurse and worked one night shift a week. I would leave my office and head to the daycare to pick them up and spend the evening and night with them. The following morning I would take her to school and him to daycare the next morning. We would go out to eat, shopping or just stay home and bum around. They lived on the third floor of their apartment building and going up the stairs was very difficult. And carrying a sleeping four-year-old up three flights of stairs wore me out. I would be out of breath by the time I reached their doorway. But, I pushed forward because I couldn't say no to Brayden.

I was tired most of the time and I developed extreme Edema. My clothes were not fitting and even my shoes were tight. I did what everyone always does and used the Internet to diagnose myself. I read about Congestive Heart Failure (CHF) and thought to myself there was no way I had CHF. I decided to fight the Edema and bought over-the-counter diuretics at Walgreens. I had gained over 40 pounds in less than a month. By the third week of December, I decided to take myself to an emergency med clinic/emergency room by my house. It was after 8 pm on December 17, 2014, and I checked into the clinic. Within two hours, I was diagnosed with Congestive Heart Failure. I was given IV Lasix and I had a Foley catheter inserted. My BNP was over 2000. I was told I was being taken by ambulance to St. Lukes Hospital for admission. The next morning I had an Echocardiogram. On Saturday, I had a Heart Catheterization which showed I had a 100% blockage and two blockages in the low 90% range. I was then told I needed triple bypass surgery. It was to take place Monday.

I notified my family and friends Thursday morning along with my employer. I had and still have a habit of not telling anyone when I was sick. I didn't tell them I was going to the clinic. Needless to say, I was given a severe lecture from my family, friends and employer. They couldn't be mad at me given my situation, but I knew I should have told them. To this day, I still am hesitant in telling anyone when something is wrong with me.

Over the weekend, I was given more IV Lasix and by the day of surgery, I had lost 40 pounds of fluid. My surgery was scheduled for Monday afternoon. I didn't have much time to think about it but knew it had to be done to save my life. I had lots of visitors and was glad to see everyone but wished that I wasn't in the hospital to give them a reason to visit me. I even had some of the "guys" from my caseload and the day program come sing Christmas carols to me. That made me feel so good.

Monday morning I was woken up at 5:30 am to prep for surgery. That was a shock as I was prepared for an afternoon surgery time. I was told the surgery had been moved up in place of other elective surgeries. I told the RN I wasn't having the surgery. I had to see my family. She told me they wait for my family to see me before my surgery. I frantically made phone calls and sent texts. I was able to contact everyone. I was able to see my mom and family. My surgery lasted over six hours and it was a success! The surgeon told my family, I was very lucky as he could see that my heart was damaged from the heart attacks and he said there was damage from another incident as well. Twenty-five percent of my heart had died during all the heart attacks.

Waking up in ICU, I felt the tubes in my body. I had one in my nose and one in my throat. I could see three tubes coming out of my chest. I looked around the room and saw machines and a nurse sitting at the end of my bed. My niece April who is a Licensed Vocational Nurse and my younger brother Aloysius were in the room with me. I was told not to move and to lay still. I knew where I was and was thinking to myself, "I hope I don't get sick from the anesthesia". I couldn't talk. I suddenly felt like I was going to vomit and did. Because of the tube in my throat, no one could immediately tell what happened. The machines began to go off and it became a madhouse in my room. I was choking on my vomit and was unable to tell anyone what was happening. I was finally able to communicate with April and Aloysius. Thankfully, the nurse used the suction and I stopped choking. After that incident, I asked for and got a small dry erase board and marker to use to communicate. If you ever have to go into the hospital, take those two items with you. When you can't communicate, it is painful to deal with and it makes you realize how lucky you are to actually be able to communicate. At that point, I thought about all the times I had made decisions for my consumers over the years who could not communicate. Or all the times we the professionals would gather as a "team" and make decisions we thought were best for the consumer. Were we really doing what they wanted? A truly humbling situation for me!

Over the next few days, I began to get my strength back. Recovery was not easy. Having the tubes in my mouth and nose meant I couldn't have anything by mouth. The pink toothettes do not help. A moist washcloth to your lips makes you thirsty. One night I was so thirsty I begged and pleaded with the RN on shift to please let me have some ice chips. He repeatedly told me no. I finally convinced him to let me have one ice chip. That was the best ice chip I have ever had in my life. Yes I know it was dangerous for me to have the ice chip but it was what I wanted. And, it made me feel so much better. I spent Christmas Day in ICU and continued to recover. The tubes in my mouth and nose came out before Christmas thankfully. Removal of the chest tubes was done before I left ICU. An RN who was six months pregnant removed them. She literally climbed into bed to remove them and it felt like they were as long as a garden hose when she removed them. That was a huge relief. I learned that you listen to the RN's instructions because the tubes would have to have been reinserted if something went wrong. I started physical therapy and was moved to a private room. I was provided a Zoll Life Vest to wear once I got home. A life vest is basically a portable defibrillator you wear under your shirt. It will literally shock your heart if something were to happen and cause your heart to stop. I left the hospital on December 28, 2014, and went to stay with Tonya and Alfred in Boerne. I was so glad to be heading home after eleven nights. I felt better leaving than I did when I went into the hospital. I had lost about 50 pounds of fluid and felt stronger.

Two days later I went grocery shopping with Tonya for their annual New Year Eve's party. I also stopped by my office to get my paycheck and say hello to everyone. I would be off work until I got my release from my doctor to return. While at the grocery store, I pushed the cart which ended up full of groceries. I ran into a friend who is an RN. We had worked together. She read me the riot act for being in public with my incision making me susceptible for infection. Of course, we had to finish shopping and did. The next day I felt like I had moved a truck. I had to rest most of the day. On New Year's Eve, I played bartender at the party making shots, serving drinks and enjoying a few myself. By 2 am I was dead tired and crashed. I slept late the following day and cleaned up after the party. Over the next few weeks, I recovered and felt better. Sleeping wasn't easy. I needed lots of help with everything. I realized that doing too much and pushing myself was not a good idea. One night we went to dinner and I used my left arm to pull myself up into my brother's F350 and I felt like I had ripped my chest open. Luckily I hadn't done so. I had no episodes of shortness of breath and I didn't have any Edema. I was weighing myself daily and I got down to 228 pounds! Prior to my heart issues, I had successfully lost over 140 pounds over a number of years and weighed 240 pounds. All the fluid retention and Edema pushed me back closer to 300 pounds. My vitals were stable and my blood pressure was low. We went to a Super Bowl party down the road and the weather was very cold. I had noticed since my heart surgery, I had gone from being hot natured to be cold natured. The party was held in a converted chicken coop that was now a large man cave. Leaving the party, I was not able to get warm. I was shivering so much that my blood pressure rose higher than it had been in a very long time. I don't recall ever having blood pressure that high. I was able to get warm and my blood pressure returned to normal. My cardiac surgeon explained that due to the amount of time my chest was open combined with the temperature of the operating room, my change in body temperature was normal.

I returned to work the beginning of February 2015 just over six weeks after having my triple bypass. I felt good and had energy again. I was able to perform my job. I did do things a little slower but was careful. Walking between buildings was not an issue and going up the stairs wasn't either. I continued to see my cardiologist and went to cardiac rehab.

I was having a lot of problems with my emotions and dealing with everything that had happened to me. People around me said I need to see a therapist. I would drive from San Antonio to Seguin every weekend to see my family. I was born and raised in Seguin and lived there most of my life. Seeing my family made me feel good despite being emotional. I was driving back home on Sunday night and KLove was on the radio. I was thinking about everything and I realized God was there to listen to me and be my therapist. I started to cry as I listened to the music. The tears flowed for almost 45 minutes as I drove. I pulled into my driveway and opened my garage door. I stopped crying and felt amazingly better. I then continued to use KLove and God as my therapy. It was very reasonable in cost and made the most sense. And, my crying didn't stop. It got better as I continued to listen to the music and allow God back into my life. I was baptized Catholic and lost touch with the church. I never lost my faith in God. It had just become extremely weak. So glad I reenergized my faith.

I wore my life vest but it was a pain in the ass. It went off several times and I was able to stop the charge. It went off while I was playing pool and once in Walmart. I had to get a smaller vest and then my skin was dry which caused the attempted shock. After a while, I stopped wearing it. Then, my cardiologist and insurance company intervened. My cardiologist recommended I see a surgeon to discuss having a pacemaker/defibrillator implanted as I wasn't wearing the life vest. My insurance company stated they would stop paying for the life vest if I didn't wear it. I returned the life vest. On October 1, 2015, I had surgery to have an ICD-D implanted in my chest near my left shoulder. The surgery was to be done, outpatient. I had to spend the night due to excessive bleeding. During the surgery, I did wake up during the surgery as the surgeon was pacing my heart to see what my heart could handle so to speak. An RN said I was in lots of pain. I heard the surgeon asking people in the room math problems related to my heart. I was answering them before they could. I said I was awake and they quickly put me back to sleep just before they made the incision. The ICD-D is a dual device meaning it is a pacemaker and defibrillator combination. The pacemaker paces my heart if it beats too fast or too slow. As my cardiologist says, it's my life insurance. Brayden calls it my superpower. He has a superpower too but don't tell him I told you so! After the surgery, I went back to work in less than a week.

In the middle of October, I had one of my guys move into the house with me. I became his foster care provider. Brian knew me well and my family loved him. He was excited and so was I. Everything was going well until I started having issues with fluid retention. My diuretic was changed twice. I played bartender again and this time, I could only stay awake until about 11:30 pm when I left the party and went inside the house and literally crashed on the bed. The next day I felt horrible and went to see my cardiologist. It was determined that all the fluid from my implant surgery had caused fluid overload. My body couldn't handle it. During that visit to the cardiologist, I learned that I had been having memory issues along with other concerns presented to my cardiologist from my boss Amy and Tonya. As the issues were being discussed I lost it. My cardiologist asked if I wanted to stop and I said no. My emotions were going wild because I couldn't believe what I was hearing because I honestly didn't know it was happening. I didn't want to believe it. I chose to be hospitalized to remove the fluid from my body. The fluid was removed and I returned back to work. I hurt my shoulder later in the year and took a lot of Ibuprofen for the pain. I developed fluid overload from taking Ibuprofen and was hospitalized from the fluid overload. Everything returned back to normal until the following year. In October 2016, I felt bad and thought I was getting the flu and strep throat. I was spitting blood and went to the ER. The wait was over 8 hours and I went back home deciding to call my cardiologist the next morning. I woke up the next morning and showered. After my shower, I passed out and woke up in a pool of blood with my head hurting. I passed out and managed to land in the doorway between my bedroom and my bathroom. I landed on the floor next to my bed. I was weak and managed to call 911 and go unlock the front door. I ended up with a hospital stay lasting over two weeks. I had developed a tear in my throat which caused the bleeding. I was close to dying had I not gotten medical treatment. Once again, I returned back to work and remained healthy until the following February when I developed an infection from an airborne illness. This time I was in the hospital for over 30 days.

I returned back to work and was told my job performance had suffered from all my hospitalizations and that I was basically no longer doing my job to the best of my abilities. I didn't argue and submitted my 30-day resignation. I didn't want to end up being terminated. At first, I felt like I had been kicked to the curb. Looking back, I understand their decision. I was always putting 110% into my job but since my heart issue started, I had lost the edge. I could play catch-up better than anyone else. But when you work with people with disabilities, they deserve 110% and I was no longer doing that. My entire 30-year career always involved putting the consumer first about all else. Sadly, I had fallen too far behind and I was doing a disservice to the guys and to my employer.

After leaving work, my stress level went down to just about zero. I talked with my Cardiologist and we discussed stress. She told me that every time I had a hospitalization the life of my heart suffered. And, stress does the same thing to my heart. I was given a life expectancy of ten years after my surgery in 2014. That number has stuck in my head but now I realize its just a number and I can live past benchmark by taking care of myself. That means keeping my stress level to a minimum. Monitoring my fluid and sodium intake. Taking my medications as ordered. Keeping my appointments as scheduled and following my doctor's orders. My ejection fraction has improved from around 20% to 40%. I no longer work and have been awarded disability. In December 2017, a foot infection resulted in the amputation of my right foot just above the ankle. I moved back home with my family and now live back in Seguin. Brian had to move in with another foster family and we continue to stay in touch. I am currently saving to get my prosthetic, as I no longer have insurance. Being in a wheelchair I have learned more about humility and patience. I look forward to the day when I get my prosthetic. In the meantime, I am volunteering at church, baking for family and friends, helping with this book and getting ready to work on recipes for people with heart disease! I am co-owner of a CHF support group online which has been a true blessing. I am staying busier than ever and I will say my heart is doing great! As my Cardiologist says, 'Keep doing what you are doing because it's obviously working.' If you do the same, you too can live with CHF and be a warrior!"

Thanks for sharing this wonderful story.

Chris Gehrke   Strawberry Plains, TN (Co-Author)

Chris has been in our CHF world for 3 years. He is the owner of a Congestive Heart Failure Support Board on Facebook.

The main symptom he experiences are explained as:

"Reduced Ejection Fraction (EF)."

CHF has impacted his quality of life described like this:

"Luckily, it hasn't affected me too much. I can still do most everything I want to physically. It has more affected me emotionally. I worry each day if it will be my last. Anytime I get a pain I'm my chest I have to worry about if it's cardiac related and if I need to go to the ER. I also know at some point it will get worse and I fear that day"

Chris is being treated with medications:

"The standard, ACE inhibitor, beta blocker, blood thinners, and cholesterol medicine. I also take depression medications.."

He is experiencing Depression/ Anxiety described like this:

"I am, but I try not to let it affect me. The main issue is the fear of not knowing what is going on in my body. I don't know if I'm getting better or worse. It is scary, but I don't let it control me. What's done is done. I just keep pushing forward."

He says the worst thing about CHF is:

"Knowing that I could die at any time. The process of dying with CHF is slow and generally not a fun process for anyone. I don't look forward to that."

This is the story she wanted to share:

"My journey isn't anything special. I eat better and try to take care of myself. I have learned to listen to my body and appreciate each day. My journey has really just begun and I hope it's a long one."

Thanks for sharing your story.

Saprina N.   Powell, OH   (#3)

Saprina has been a CHF patient battling it for 3 years.

The main symptoms she experiences are:

"Shortness of breath, dizziness, pain, Edema, weight gain, fatigue, exercise intolerance, anxiety, depression, hard time sleeping, nausea and syncope."

CHF has impacted her quality of life. She explained it this way:

"Hard to complete daily tasks, can no longer work, rarely have energy for socializing, rely heavily on others to do things I used to do easily like grocery shopping. Have loads of anxiety now. Very little sleep. It has affected relationships quality of life is not good."

The medications she is taking are:

"Blood pressure meds, vasodilators, ARB, depression meds, anxiety meds, diuretics, ACE inhibitors, sleep meds and GERD meds."

She is experiencing Depression described like this:

"The frustration of not being able to do the things I use to do. Fear of falling or passing out. Being alone when something happens. Not being treated for pain."

She feels the worst thing about CHF is:

"The loss of self"

This is the story she wanted to share:

"The journey has taught me many things about myself and my loved ones. Unless you are going through it, it is hard to make people understand your limitations. It's like a box of chocolates, you never know what kind of day you are going to have good, bad or barely hanging on."

Thanks for sharing this story.

Name Withheld Fort Worth, TX   (#4)

This Member has just entered the CHF world and has had the illness for 11 months.

The main symptoms being experienced are:

"Memory loss, random smells out of nowhere and weight gain."

CHF has only made a minor impacted quality of life. As explained this way:

"I had to get an ICD, but can still maintain an excellent quality of life. I exercise, I try to eat right. Other than getting tired more quickly I don't notice a change. I'm lucky so far."

The medications the member is being treated with are:

"Lasix, Metoprolol, Losartan and baby aspirin."

The member is experiencing Depression and anxiety described this way:

"I had major anxiety and slight depression before the diagnosis. Both still are issues but being a single mother, I can't let it get me down. I'm afraid of dying so I bury my head in the sand and push on through."

The member feels the worst thing about CHF is:

"The fear of the not knowing what's going to happen."

This is the story they wanted to share:

"I went to the dentist with a broken tooth and they pulled it. I am prone to infection and got one and it made me sick. Move forward about two months and I went to ER thinking I had severe bronchitis and they said CHF. It's been a roller coaster ever since. I'm in Texas, my family is in Missouri. This roller coaster is very scary when you are alone with just your children. Add on an emotionally abusive ex-husband and his witch of a live-in girlfriend that is horrible to your kids, makes it tough. But again, I try not to question God too much and push through. It gets hard sometimes but I can't let it get me down for my boys."

Thanks for sharing this story.

Kelly R.   Milton, TN (#5)

Kelly is fairly new to the CHF battle and has had it for 3 months.

The main symptoms being experienced are:

"Weight gain, shortness of breath, Edema, chest pain and dizziness."

CHF has made a definite impacted on quality of life. As explained this way:

"CHF has had a huge impact on my life! I was extremely active and now struggle to do just the basics in life."

The meds Kelly is being treated with include this:

"20 pills a day plus 2 inhalers. Also taking B12 shots weekly and Cosentyx shot every 14 days."

Kelly is experiencing Depression and anxiety described like this:

"I get depressed because I can't do the things I use to enjoy doing. My family treats me as if I am so fragile that I'll break. I have anxiety that keeps me from trying to push myself."

Kelly feels the worst thing about CHF is:

"Shortness of breath and fatigue."

This is the story she wanted to share:

"I come from a family of people who drop dead from heart attacks. I've been having palpitations for about 5 years. I started seeing my cardiologist about the palpitations. They ran every kind of test and my heart always checked out ok. Then at the beginning of the year I was short of breath and had a horrible cough but didn't feel sick. I saw my PCP and she treated me for pneumonia. After antibiotics, I was still short of breath so she treated me again and set up an appointment with the Pulmonary Lab at Vanderbilt. By the time of my appointment, I could only walk about 10 ft before wheezing and coughing trying to catch my breath. I passed the pulmonary test. Then the pulmonologist came in to tell me how I did on the test and he showed me all of the heart tests and lung scans and told me I have Diastolic Heart Dysfunction and Diastolic Heart Failure. I was shocked! I started googling stuff and everything said 10-year life expectancy! I gave the news to my family. Then I found the wonderful support group on FB where people have been living with CHF for 30 years! That gave me so much hope!! With my medications and watching my diet, I am doing much better. I still can't clean my house or do a whole lot but I am doing ok. I even made it to the gym today! There is hope!"

Thanks for sharing this story.

Al S.   *Nacogdoches, TX*   *(#6)*

Al has been in the CHF battle for 2 years.

The main symptoms being experienced are:

"Edema, shortness of breath, chest pain, memory loss and frequent falls."

CHF has made an impacted on his quality of life. As explained this way:

"I am unable to work, unable to spend play time with my kids, unable to sleep and a lot of pain."

The meds he is being treated with include this:

"A very long list of cardiac medication, fluid pills, pain pills, blood thinners."

Al is experiencing depression and anxiety and described it like this:

"Anxiety because I know the time will come that my heart can no longer work and this alone is freaking me out."

The worst thing about CHF is:

"The daily battle to stay alive. I take so many pills that I am not even hungry for food. The happiness that this condition has taken from me."

This is the story he wanted to share:

"I am 45 years old Ex police officer and paramedic and I have end stage heart failure. Because of this condition, I have to file for bankruptcy, lost time with my family and I have lost friends. This condition was unexpected. I was diagnosed with CHF after by triple bypass surgery but I continued to work. March of 2018, I went into VFIB and after they brought me back, my cardiologist decided that I get an ICD. After this my EF was at 23% so I was not allowed to return to work. Since these two skills are all I have I have filled for disability. Still waiting on SSDI to approve me. This month alone I have fallen three times so my doctor ordered me a wheelchair. Also, my kidneys are beginning to fail me."

Thanks for sharing this story.

Jackie   *Jeannette, PA*   *(#7)*

Jackie has been a CHF patient battling for 2 years.

The main symptoms she experiences are:

"Weight gain, severe fatigue, light headed, swell in the stomach."

CHF has impacted her quality of life. She explained it this way:

"It has changed my life tremendously. I have cardiomyopathy/chef from a chemo drug doxorubicin aka red devil. I am a survivor of Non-Hodgkin's my quality of life is very poor. I struggle to do just activities of daily living. I can't walk far or do anything I previously enjoyed."

The medications she is taking are:

"Coreg, Irbesartan, Magnesium, Vitamin D, Lasix and COq10."

She is experiencing Depression described like this:

"Yes, I am severely depressed being unable to do the things I could before. Not being able to do much with my family feel like a burden and am unable to work."

She says the worst thing about CHF is:

"For me the fatigue"

This is the story she wanted to share:

"Nine years ago, I had a 38 by 34 tumor around my heart. Did chemo with Doxorubicin then went back to work long hours and thought I was tired. Apparently, a few years later I was in moderate heart failure from the drug and by 2016 I was struggling to carry groceries and climbing the stairs. At 38 years old and after a long battle with cancer this has been a long road most of my family is passed on and I have a daughter and struggle with support and feel as though I am sleeping my life away I am being told that a heart transplant is my only option but the chances of getting on the list may not be possible because of having had the Non-Hodgkin's and also unsure if my body would be able to handle anti-rejection drugs after 2 years on the medications I am on, my ejection fraction has not progressed at all"

Thanks for sharing this story.

Starla L.   *Sierra Vista, AZ (#8)*

Starla has been a CHF patient for 4 years.

The main symptoms she experiences are:

"Weight gain, Edema, memory loss, dizziness, lightheadedness and fainting."

CHF has impacted her quality of life. She explained it this way:

"I went from supermom of 4 who was a Girl Scout leader, ran an in-home daycare, football team mom, baseball team mom, and homeschooled 3 children to a couch potato that depends on my children's help."

The medications she is taking are:

"Entresto, Allopurinol, Spironolactone, Coreg, Torsemide, aspirin, 2 inhalers, breathing treatments, potassium, iron, vitamin d, antidepressants and Montelukast."

She is experiencing Depression/ Anxiety described like this:

"Yes, I have anxiety from fear of others judgements and fainting at stores or business while out. I'm depressed because I feel like I have had my life, hopes, and dreams stolen."

She says the worst thing about CHF is:

"Not looking as sick as I am and struggling to breathe"

This is the story she wanted to share:

"I was a vegan who ran a mile 3 times a week when out of nowhere my hands and feet started to swell. I went from a diagnosis of left bundle branch block and congestive heart failure with an ejection fraction of 45 in April 2014 to having open heart surgery to replace my aortic valve and stem and getting a pacemaker due to an ejection fraction of 35 and complete heart block in June 2014."

Thanks for sharing this story.

Sheila F.   Waldorf, MD   (#9)

Sheila is pretty new to CHF as a patient for 8 months.

The main symptoms she experiences are:

"Shortness of breath, dizziness and extended abdomen."

CHF has impacted her quality of life. She explained it this way:

"I'm not as active as I was. My CHF was due to Scleroderma and I'm on oxygen."

The medications she is taking are:

"Ramipril, Carvedilol and Cellcept."

She is experiencing Depression/ Anxiety described like this:

"Yes, I do. The quality of life because I have other health issues. I got fired from my job because of my illness and I feel like I don't contribute to the household because I'm not working. I have sought help for my depression and I'm on mild anti-anxiety meds, it helps."

She says the worst thing about CHF is:

"Not knowing what tomorrow may bring."

This is the story she wanted to share:

"My story starts with my Scleroderma diagnosis in 2010 and I have been dealing with severe lung and muscle disease. The CHF came out of nowhere because I never had the typical symptoms it was caught by chance during a Cath for my lungs. I'm still trying to wrap my head around it."

Thanks for sharing this story.

Name Withheld   Raleigh, NC   (#10)

This member has been in the CHF battle for two and a half years.

The main symptoms they experience are:

"Occasional dizziness, weight gain, slight memory loss, out of breath quickly with strenuous exercise."

CHF has impacted their quality of life. They explained it this way:

"Cannot do some hobbies I enjoy, no longer travel to 3rd world countries, must be very careful with my diet and because of that, miss foods I enjoyed."

The medications they are taking are:

"Beta blocker, ACE inhibitor, loop diuretic, potassium sparing diuretic, statin, antiplatelet, 325mg aspirin, Pepcid, Magnesium, CoQ10, fish oil, multivitamin."

They are <u>not</u> experiencing Depression/ Anxiety.

They say the worst thing about CHF is:

"Not being able to participate in some sports and hobbies and anticipating an eventual decline in my condition."

This is the story they wanted to share:

"I had a massive MI in April of 2016, with lots of damage. My ejection fraction was 20%. In July of that year, I was hospitalized with flash pulmonary Edema & pleural effusion (fluid on the outside of my lungs). While in the hospital a scan revealed "enlarged lymph tissue" in my upper thorax......sounds similar to your enlarged nodules. My pulmonologist started watching that enlarged lymph tissue, & it was not receding. Also, my pleural effusion was returning. She sent me to a thoracic surgeon who said he could biopsy the lymph tissue & also repaired my lungs so the pleural effusion would not return. If I had lymphoma, the treatments were all chemo, & lymphoma chemo drugs are hard on the heart & often cause heart failure, & I already had heart failure. Things were not looking good. The surgeon got in there & I did not have lymphoma, but rather, I had a tumor growing on my thymus gland, a thymoma. It's pretty rare. The surgeon removed it cleanly. The pathology came back with the best news I could have hoped for; class A, stage 1, essentially benign at that stage. I needed no chemo, & have semiannual scans now, all of which have remained clean. My surgeon says I have a 99% chance of never having a recurrence. I still have a hard time reconciling that had I not had such a bad heart attack with the resulting heart failure, I never would have known that I had the tumor & the tumor would have eventually metastasized and likely killed me. MI was a wakeup call, and I have completely changed what I eat (Ornis), and do now exercise religiously, and do take all my meds when I am supposed to, and do now follow all my doctors' instructions, and use my CPAP every day, and keep my sodium intake to <1500 mg/day, and weigh every day, and record my BP twice a day, and record my blood oxygen level twice a day, and listen to my body, and rest when I need to, and get enough sleep, and I have reduced my stress. And despite an ejection fraction of ~30%, it seems to be working, as my symptoms of heart failure are minimal and livable. My heart failure doc has for now excluded me from clinical studies because I am currently "too healthy". I am largely asymptomatic though I do have to stay on top of occasional overnight weight gain because of fluid retention. But I am

beyond grateful for having a 2nd chance at life and no longer take my health for granted."

Lois F. St. Andrews, Manitoba, Canada (#11)

Lois is an experienced CHF patient and has been in the battle for 20 years.

The main symptoms Lois experiences are:

"Edema, fatigue, dizziness, pain in legs a lot and feeling of choking."

CHF has impacted this member's quality of life who explained it this way:

"Until recently I was able to keep up pretty well, but for last couple years, I have been unable to keep up and get around much more slowly. I am really trying to keep my strength up but it is really difficult."

The medications Lois is taking are:

"Omeprazole, Warfarin, Bisoprolol. I am waiting for echo to show what else may be helpful. I was a long-time user of Celebrex but quit that a couple weeks ago per doctor's recommendations."

Lois is not experiencing Depression/ Anxiety described this way:

"No mentally I am ok. Main issue is fatigue and fluid retention.."

Lois says the worst thing about CHF is:

"I feel so lazy and just watch things pile up with no energy to deal with it. I have tired eyes and yawn all the time. I often feel that my fun life is over."

This is the story Lois wanted to share:

"I had rheumatic fever when I was 20 and damaged mitral valve. but was able to have a child and lead an active life with skiing and hiking and canoeing. In 2007 I had a valvuloplasty to stretch mitral valve which was successful and good till 2015 with another attempt to stretch out valve but I started into atrial fib afterwards."

Thanks for sharing this story.

Krystal B.   Shreveport, LA   (#12)

Krystal is new to CHF as a patient for 1 year.

The main symptoms she experiences are:

"Confusion, fluid retention and feeling weak."

CHF has impacted her quality of life. She explained it this way:

"It's turned my life around completely. I know value life."

The medications she is taking are:

"Losartan Metoprolol, Synthroid, Lasix and Spironolactone."

She is experiencing Depression/ Anxiety described like this:

"Yes, but I'm on Buspirone and it really helps."

She says the worst thing about CHF is:

"The diagnosis itself."

This is the story she wanted to share:

No story provided

Thanks for sharing this information.

Jeff V.   *Farmington, AR (#13)*

Jeff is a more experienced CHF fighter who has had it for 14 years.

The main symptoms he experiences are explained this way:

"I have experienced Edema... weight gain, fatigue, organ and muscle deterioration, dizziness with exertion, transient pain and depression, but the most remarkable thing I've suffered from is the fact that I will die much sooner than I should because I am poor. The medicines, treatments and procedures that are not covered by Medicare are not considered. If your poor you just ... die"

CHF has impacted his quality of life. He explained it this way:

"I am an honorably discharged veteran that worked 20+ years in the medical field. I raised 4 good citizens and was forced retired in 2004. The doctor actually told me I would die within 2 years, that really messed me up psychologically. I changed my diet and lifestyle to help me survive. I did all I could to extend my life. I am not able to get an LVAD or transplant due to cost and my ejection fraction is now below 20%... yea... I deal with the thought of death daily... that in itself is devastating to my life energy. I turned my life around completely. I know the value of life."

The medications he is taking are:

"Entresto (samples because it's $800.00 a month) Coreg...Spironolactone... Furosemide... and varied meds to alleviate pain associated with joint and muscle aches due to decreased nourishment from

blood... aspirin and Tylenol... I do not take opiates or narcotics due to motility issues."

He is experiencing Depression/ Anxiety described like this:

"Death is depressing... it gives you anxiety... it makes you sick with worry at times... it is not easy KNOWING your dying at a faster rate... yea... not a good feeling when your headed to the hospital for breathing issues... my biggest fear is that trip to the hospital that they don't let you leave... and you wait to die."

He says the worst thing about CHF is:

"Decreased activity with loved ones and the fact that they are watching you get sicker... not healthy for their psyche either."

This is the story he wanted to share:

"Not much of a story other than I did everything that a good citizen does... graduated school... attended college... served honorably in the military... married and raised a family for 20 years until we broke up due to my sickness... I eventually remarried and am simply trying to live and love each day that's left... it's unfortunate... but life is not perfect... simply living life as full as possible... writing down your thoughts... and hugging... that's the secret to living with a death sentence like cardiomyopathy and CHF... it's all you can do... the greatest thing I hope to accomplish at this point is simply to be fondly remembered...."

Name Withheld   *Roanoke, VA*   *(#14)*

This member has been a CHF fighter for 4 years.

The main symptoms they experience are explained this way:

"Breathing, chest pains, dizziness...light headed, fluid overload, no energy & tiredness."

CHF has impacted their quality of life. They explained it this way:

"Not being able to do 100% of what I use to do. Simple task sometimes zaps the energy out."

The medications they are taking are:

BP meds, Lasix etc. Am also end stage kidney failure 6% kidney function...so have meds to keep whatever peritoneal dialysis drains out of me.

They are experiencing Depression/ Anxiety described like this:

"Yes. Emotional roller coaster :-(."

They say the worst thing about CHF is:

"Basically, not being able to do the things I did at 100% before CHF took a hold of my life."

This is the story they wanted to share:

"Stopped breathing 4yrs ago & that is when I was diagnosed with CHF. They needed to do a heart cath., that is when I found out my kidneys were already stage 4 failure. My EF was at 15%. They found 4 blockages so had bypass. 4yrs later my EF is at 50%. My doctors concerned with lower chambers not pumping as well but that's from all the "beating" my heart has taken. Just need to concentrate on getting a kidney replacement so my heart has a "partner" & not work as hard to keep me going strong. :) They say diabetes was my main culprit for a bad heart & kidneys. Any diabetics out there need to really take that disease seriously because yes it does damage the other organs."

Thanks for sharing this story.

Sara T.   *Muncie, IN(#15)*

Sara thinks she has had CHF for 5+ years, but was only diagnosed 4 months ago

The main symptoms she experiences are explained this way:

"Low blood pressure, dizziness, fatigue, Edema, rapid heart rate."

CHF has impacted her quality of life. She explained it this way:

"Can no longer work. It is hard to make plans, because my body doesn't always cooperate"

The medications she is taking are explained this way:

"My doctor has taken me off of everything except Coreg because I can't maintain my blood pressure on the other cardiac meds. The one I notice the most change is not taking Lasix. My Edema is getting worse. I am being referred for pacemaker/defibrillator placement soon."

She is experiencing Depression/ Anxiety described like this:

"Both, I am losing my home because I can't work, have been denied disability and don't have an income, therefore cannot pay my mortgage."

She says the worst thing about CHF is:

"Not being able to do normal everyday activities anymore."

This is the story she wanted to share:

"I had a stroke in 2013. The neurologist ordered an echo when I was in the ICU. A cardiologist read it and determined I had CHF which was a causative factor in my stroke. No one told me for 5 years that I was in heart failure. I needed surgery on my shoulder, but before I scheduled it, I asked my orthopedic surgeon for a cardiology referral. I had blood work and an echo and showed stage 3 heart failure. When I had my stroke, I was in stage 1 heart failure. The cardiologist said that my hospital's rules are if a secondary discipline is not invited onto your case by the primary physicians, they cannot inform you of any medical conditions. Unfortunately, neither did my neurologist or my primary care physician after I was discharged from the hospital."

Thanks for sharing this story.

Amy M.   Macon, GA (#16)

Amy has been fighting CHF for 3 years.

The main symptoms she experiences are explained this way:

"Edema, tired, dizziness, depression."

CHF has impacted her quality of life. She explained it this way:

"CHF has changed my life completely, I feel like I'm missing the other 1/2 of me. I'm not complete. So many things that I can no longer do the simplest things"

The medications she is taking were not provided.

She is experiencing Depression/ Anxiety described like this:

"Yes, I went from a full-time job, softball mom, going no stop to making myself get out of bed before 4 pm... it's really sad."

She says the worst thing about CHF is:

"Life changes ... all of them."

This is the story she wanted to share:

"I'm a 40 year woman with a EF of 11, I have a ICD, I can no longer work , sometimes not drive. I can't stay in the heat for more the 5 min . I take 22 pills a day .. lost most of my Friends because they don't understand .. Because I don't LOOK SICK. It's hard for my kids to understand and sometimes my husband and mine was a case of bad luck. I've never had a heart attack .. no blockages ..not really over weight. I exercised and watch what I ate, but a little over 3 year ago I had the flu and it attacked my heart it was viral. It started off with weight gain, couldn't breath, had to rest when taking short walks. I went to the doctor, sent me to a Cardiologist and now I have Cardiomyopathy."

Thanks for sharing this story.

Gillian M.   Abbots Langley, Herts, UK   (#17)

Gillian has been fighting in the CHF world for 5 years.

The main symptoms she experiences are explained this way:

"Edema, breathlessness and tiredness."

CHF has impacted her quality of life. She explained it this way:

"Have to pace myself as I tire easily."

The medications she is taking is:

"Betablockers, anti-hypertensives, statins, aspirin and Spironolactone ."

She is not experiencing Depression/ Anxiety from her CHF.

She says the worst thing about CHF is:

"Tiredness leading to complete exhaustion."

She did not share an individual story.
Thanks for sharing this information.

Reuben J.   Topeka, KS   (#18)

Reuben has been fighting CHF in our world for 6 years.

The main symptoms he experiences are explained this way:

"Water weight, dizziness, slight chest pains, sweating, body feeling drained, tired, lack of sleep, coughing, low blood pressure. Please note that some of these could be from the medications I take in upwards of 14 pills a day, some taken twice."

CHF has impacted his quality of life. He explained it this way:

"A huge impact some due to my age and having a family. The loss of income, taking its toll on relationships and less social interactions."

The medications he is taking are:

"Fourteen or more different meds ranging from a constant IV to pills, some are precautionary some are needed such as the dieretic, blood thinner and blood pressure."

He is experiencing Depression/ Anxiety described like this:

"I am sure, I have some to a degree but I manage to get by. The biggest one is stress it usually wears me down."

He says the worst thing about CHF is:

_____

"The possible outcome."

_____

This is the story he wanted to share:

_____

"I found out on my 35th birthday, life changed from then on. I no longer work and it took its toll on my marriage after 3 years. Most of my time is spent with my family and friends. Every day is a battle that I will continue to fight.

_____

Thanks for sharing this story.

Joy   *North Carolina*   *(#19)*

Joy is pretty new to the world of CHF and has only had it for 1 year.

The main symptoms she experiences are explained this way:

"Edema, dizziness and insomnia."

CHF has impacted her quality of life. She explained it this way:

"It has changed my future plans. I have to adapt to not having much energy."

She is being treated with these medications:

"Entresto, Lasix, Coreg, Atorvastatin, Aspirin, Spironolactone and Janumet. Co Q 10, and Vit. B"

She is not experiencing Depression/ Anxiety.

She says the worst thing about CHF is:

"Loss of energy."

This is the story she wanted to share:

"I had a silent MI, December 2017. Found to have CHF at that time. Taken to the Cath lab, found no significant blockages. EF was 23%. Put on meds, EF has risen to 40%. Also have SVT, may need cardioversion in future."

Thanks for sharing this story.

Darren W.   Columbia, SC   (#20)

Darren is another of our very experienced patients having CHF for 30 years.

The main symptoms he experiences are explained this way:

"No regular symptoms only side effects from medications."

CHF has impacted his quality of life. He explained it this way:

"Fear and anxiety. Scared for my future and financial burdens from medical bills."

Darren is being treated with the following medications:

"Metoprolol, Sotalol, Lisinopril and baby aspirin."

He is experiencing Depression/ Anxiety described like this:

"Yes both, fear of the medical cost and not being alive and leaving behind my wife, daughter and family."

He says the worst thing about CHF is:

"Not being able to do all the things I would like to do."

This is the story he wanted to share:

"I am 32 years old. I was born with CAD (Coronary Artery Disease), it went undiagnosed at birth. When I was 18 months old I had a heart attack. my heart was repaired but damage was done. My EF has been 30-35% my entire life. I have an ICD implant and suffer from VTAC due to the scar tissue on my left ventricle, as a result of my heart attack. I have had CHF since being a child and was told I needed a heart transplant by the time I would turn 16. I have yet to need the transplant and live a normal life. When I was 18. I started to have episodes of VTAC and continue to.".

Thanks for sharing this story.

Jen D.   Hawley, PA   (#21)

Jen has been in the CHF battle for 5 years.

The main symptoms she experiences are explained this way:

"SOB, chest pain and fatigue."

CHF has impacted her quality of life. She explained it this way:

"I have to stay in the air conditioning in my bedroom. I can't breathe in the hot humid summer air. I miss gardening and the beach."

Jen is being treated with the following medications:

"Entresto, Aspirin, Metoprolol, Amlodipine, Nephrovite, Atorvastatin, Xanax, calcium acetate, Veltessa."

She is experiencing Depression/ Anxiety described like this:

"I think I suffer from depression at times. I miss my old life before I was sick."

She says the worst thing about CHF is:

"The sudden buildup of fluid that makes it hard to breathe."

This is the story she wanted to share:

"I had a heart attack and my kidneys failed due to uncontrolled high blood pressure. I have been fighting both diseases for 5 years now. It's scary and exhausting.

Thanks for sharing this story.

Kathy M.   *Mentor, OH*   (#22)

Kathy is experienced and has been in the CHF battle for 18 years.

The main symptoms she experiences are explained this way:

"No significant symptoms. Mild palpitations on occasion. Anxiety."

CHF has impacted her quality of life. She explained it this way:

"Since ICD implant no impact."

Kathy is being treated with the following medications:

"Coreg, Spironolactone and Valsartan."

She is not experiencing significant Depression/ Anxiety.

She says the worst thing about CHF is:

"Having a condition that could shorten my life."

This is the story she wanted to share:

"My heart was damaged following Chemo for breast cancer. I have survived 18 years. Took a while to feel good enough to enjoy travel and grandchildren."

Thanks for sharing this story.

Kim M. Trumann, AR (#23)

Kim is pretty new to the CHF battle and has had it for 9 months.

The main symptom she experiences is "*Fatigue*".

CHF has impacted her quality of life. She explained it this way:

"I get tired quicker but it made me appreciate life more. I am living more now than before."

Kim is being treated with the following medications:

"I take over 12 each day, including Entresto, Eliquis, Coreg, Jardiance, Lasix, Spironolactone, Metformin, Glipizide, insulin."

She is experiencing Depression/ Anxiety described like this:

"I have anxiety and take Buspar for it."

She says the worst thing about CHF is:

"Worrying about dying."

She did not choose to share a story.

Antony W. Swindon, Wiltshire, UK   (#24)

Antony has been in the CHF battle for 2 years.

The main symptoms he experiences are explained this way:

"Edema, breathlessness and dizziness."

CHF has impacted his quality of life. He explained it this way:

"Had to retire from work."

Antony's comment about medications:

"Too many to mention (17)."

He is experiencing Depression/ Anxiety described like this:

"Frustrated at not being able to do what I used to do."

He did not choose to say the worst thing about CHF or to share his life story.

Name Withheld Harrisburg, PA   (#25)

This member has been in the CHF battle for a little over a year.

The main symptoms they experience are explained this way:

"SOB and tiredness."

CHF has impacted their quality of life. They explained it this way:

"Had to severely limit volunteer activities, gardening and shopping."

They are being treated with the following medications:

"Coreg, Vasotec and Aldactone."

They are experiencing Depression/ Anxiety described like this:

"Anxiety about possibility of getting an ICD."

They say the worst thing about CHF is:

"Being tired and SOB. Not knowing how much worse CHF will get and not entirely trusting doctors and other medical staff!"

This is the story they wanted to share:

"I have had HBP and LBBB for years. In the summer of 2016, I began to have heart palpitations, which I had had before off and on, but I finally mentioned them to my PCP. Months later, he made a referral to a cardiologist. I was diagnosed with PVCs---no big problem. Then I got a bad cold and bronchitis and coughed for months. When I finally recovered from the bronchitis and scheduled the Echocardiogram, my EF had dropped from over 50% four years ago to 20% in March 2017. When I finally got to see the Cardiologist in June 2017, he diagnosed Dilated Cardiomyopathy, started Coreg and immediately started pushing PM/ICD. (My mother was diagnosed with dilated cardiomyopathy at age 90 and had a PM.) No diet restrictions or exercise even mentioned or recommended by my Cardiologists. After the Coreg was doubled a month later, I got really, really ill and was diagnosed with Acute on Chronic CHF. Lasix prescribed and EF decreased to 15% in September 2017. I had little improvement over several months. I stayed indoors except for necessary grocery shopping and doctor's appointments for months because of the fear of catching the flu. Tried Entresto for a few months, then discontinued due to tiredness. In March 2018, on my own I started doing breathing exercises and walking. I requested a referral to the Heart Failure Clinic because I felt I was not getting adequate information from my doctors. I found Clinic visits very helpful and was angry that I had not been referred there by any one of the three doctors I had seen over the last year! I found online support groups very helpful. I feel much better now and am currently trying to raise my EF to at least 35% through diet, exercise and meds because I will not consent to an ICD unless I am flat on my back in the hospital! Pacemaker---maybe, if I am presented with actual evidence/studies that it is needed and will improve the quality of my life. I walk about a mile most days and can log up to 2.5 miles a day while shopping and gardening. I am 75 years old and in very good health, otherwise.

Jeff S.   *Gatlinburg, TN*   (#26)

Jeff has been in the CHF world for 4 years.

The main symptoms he experiences are explained this way:

"Depression, Fluid buildup, Loss of energy, Dizziness, Social Anxiety... since I'm home alone most of the time, Pain and Always cold"

CHF has impacted his quality of life. He explained it this way:

"It's practically slowed me down to turtle speed."

Jeff is being treated with the following medications:

"Xarelto, Coreg, Bumex, Spironolactone, Xanax, potassium and Lisinopril."

He is experiencing Depression/ Anxiety described like this:

"That's the million-dollar question. Since my diagnosis. I have tried to hurt myself thru attempted suicide, I now have social anxiety, and I've began to have delusions of things and people that aren't there.

He says the worst thing about CHF is:

"I feel pretty useless"

This is the story he wanted to share:

"I was diagnosed with CHF 4 years ago. On 4 separate occasions I have been admitted to the hospital for severe fluid retention. All over 100 lbs. The most was 172 lbs. of fluid. My legs were so swollen from the fluid the skin was cracking. I was there for over a month and was sent to a rehabilitation nursing home. For 1 month. Now I'm suffering from depression, social anxiety, and starting to have delusions. Situations like, talking and having conversations that never ever happened. Some paranoia. I'm now homebound and never have any friends over and family doesn't ever visit."

Thanks for sharing this story.

Christina S.   Lakewood, CO   (#27)

Christina is a fairly new addition to the CHF world and has had it for about 1 year.

The main symptoms she experiences are explained this way:

"Edema, weight gain, dizziness, pain, shortness of breath, chest pain, low blood pressure, PVCs and dehydration"

CHF has impacted her quality of life. She explained it this way:

"I was unable to work the first 4 months after my diagnosis. I have missed a lot of work due to my illness which caused me to almost lose my job. My husband and I have separated twice because he can't handle what's going on. We are currently separated. We have a 2-year-old daughter and it's been very difficult to play and do fun activities with her since I'm tired a lot. My EF started out at 14% in July 2017 and by October 2017 it was at 40%. I had an echo July 2018 and it's still at 40% with no improvement. I also have Dilatated Cardiomyopathy and have had no change in the dilation of my heart. I have had one rough year."

Christina is being treated with the following medications:

"Beta blocker, ace inhibitor, Lasix, potassium sparing diuretic, thyroid, depression, potassium and a multi vitamin."

She is experiencing Depression/ Anxiety described like this:

"Yes, I am suffering from depression currently. When I first went back to work I was having really bad anxiety, but not as much anymore. I have fatigue which makes me just want to sleep or lie around. I'm not motivated to work out or even get out of the house. I feel very down a lot and sad."

She says the worst thing about CHF is:

"The worst thing is how it's effected my daughter. I've had to put her through a lot the past year."

This is the story she wanted to share:

"In April 2017 I began having chest pain and right sided pain. Because the pain was more on my right side I immediately thought it was my gall bladder. I was seen by my doctor who sent me for an ultrasound which did not show anything. A week later the pain was worse and I had a fever and my pulse was racing. I went to the ER and they checked my gallbladder again and nothing. So, they diagnosed me with an ulcer and sent me home. I soon developed a really bad virus and a horrible cough that wouldn't go away. I still had the cough a month later and the pain was back. My doctor ordered an endoscopy to be done. I had the scope done and they found nothing. It was now July and I was still having pain my cough was still there. The pain was bad but now I was having shortness of breath and a racing heart. I work in surgery and was in a lot of pain and a doctor I work with advised me to go to the ER. I went and the ultra sound now showed an inflamed gall bladder. I had my gall bladder out the next day and the pain was gone so I thought. Two days later I woke up and my stomach was bruised and swollen. I thought it was due to the air they put in my abdomen during surgery. I went in 5 days after surgery and was extremely swollen mostly in my abdomen. My heart rate was really high I

was having chest and abdominal pain and shortness of breath. I was admitted as soon as I was seen in my surgeon's office. I was immediately sent for a CT scan which determined I had Edema. By the end of the night I was diagnosed with Dilated Cardiomyopathy and told I was in heart failure with an EF of 14%. I was in the hospital 5 days where I lost 27 pounds of fluid. I was sent home with a life vest that I wore for 3 months. I had an Echo done in October 2017 and my EF was up to 40%. I went back to work 1-2 days a week the first 2 months then finally back full time at the beginning of 2018. I have had good and bad days and many trips to the urgent care and ER. I had an echo at one year in July 2018 which showed no change since October. Every day is a struggle. I'm not sure if I'll feel good when I wake up the next day."

Thanks for sharing this story.

Sue J.   Wellston, OH   (#28)

Sue is a newer addition to the CHF world and has had it for about 1 year.

The main symptoms she experiences are explained this way:

"Short of breath and chest pain"

CHF has impacted her quality of life. She explained it this way:

"Had to quit coaching, kept me close to home for 6 months."

Sue is being treated with the following medications:

"Two blood pressure meds, a nitrate, water pill, cholesterol, baby aspirin and potassium."

She is experiencing Depression/ Anxiety described like this:

"Mornings spent in bathroom!! Depression early on, not now. Diet makes it hard to go out and just enjoy myself."

She says the worst thing about CHF is:

"Getting tired so quickly."

This is the story she wanted to share:

"Bladder issues was how it began. Treated for over a year with the wrong diagnosis. Shortness of breath and chest pain followed. Stopped working as a substitute teacher because of it. Went in for a Catherization and was told I had CHF and not a blockage. Sent to heart failure MD. With strict diet and correct meds as well as many calls to the cardiac nurse, things are better. I am thankful."

Thanks for sharing this story.

Carol C.   Lockwood, NY   (#29)

Carol is a new addition to the CHF world and has had it for almost 1 year.

The main symptoms she experiences are explained this way:

"Edema and shortness of breath"

CHF has impacted her quality of life by making her, *"mostly homebound"*.

Carol is being treated with the following medications:

"Lasix, Spironolactone, Entresto, Corlanor, Plavix and Eliquis."

She is experiencing Depression/ Anxiety described like this:

"Take Venlafaxine for depression and Alprazolam infrequently for anxiety. Slows me down very much."

She says the worst thing about CHF is:

"Shortness of breath after walking only 10 feet or less. Steps are almost impossible."

This is the story she wanted to share:

" Started in 2000 with open heart for two blockages. April 2011, mitral valve replacement via open heart. 2016 blood clot on mitral valve. 2017 in hospital seven times for various heart issues and stents. January 2018, respiratory arrest and intubation followed by heart attack with very high troponin levels. Went to inpatient rehab wearing a Life Vest. Had this until March when it defibrillated me for VTAC. Cardiologist inserted an Automatic Implanted Defibrillator and pacemaker. Added above meds. No beta blockers make breathing worse. Now home almost six months doing well.

Thanks for sharing this story.

Dixie C.   St. John, NB, Canada   (#30)

Dixie has been in the CHF world for 2 years.

The main symptoms she experiences are explained this way:

"Pain., shortness of breath, dizziness and swelling"

CHF has impacted her quality of life by, *"limitations"*.

Dixie is being treated with the following medication:

"Entresto".

She is experiencing Depression/ Anxiety.

She says the worst thing about CHF is:

"No one understands.... isolation."

This is the story she wanted to share:

"I am a 62 female ... I never give in or up. I have had 3 heart attacks, 30 stents, ejection factor of 25%... triple bypass, AAA 4.1 cm enlarged heart, 6 trips to Cath lab... 3 existing critical blockages which cannot be fixed with a stint. I live my life to the fullest everyday."

Lisa W. Ogden, UT (#31)

Lisa has been in the CHF world for 3 years.

The main symptoms she experiences are explained this way:

"Shortness of breath, swollen legs (pitting Edema), tiredness, lightheadedness, and didn't feel good"

CHF has impacted her quality of life described like this:

"It changed it. Before I was diagnosed I'd began to feel a gradual decline — I couldn't do the things I normally did. I got very tired easily. My 40 hrs. plus at work in a call center went down to 4 days then to 3 because I just couldn't do it anymore. I'd come home and had no life because I just wanted to sit. It also took a toll on family because I didn't have the energy to work, take care of house cleaning, cooking meals, cleaning up etc. I was eventually let go of that job (end of season) but had troubles doing another job because I couldn't get out and work with people. I'd be so short of breath just walking from the car sometimes. I later started another job as a cashier which lasted about 3 months I just couldn't keep up and by then I'd had a heart catheterization and my doctor told me to file for disability not to work anymore."

Lisa is being treated with medications:

"I am on diuretics first started out with hydrochlorothiazide. Then was changed to Furosemide and Spironolactone was added now I am on Torsemide and Spironolactone also take Propafenone, Metoprolol, potassium and Eliquis"

She is experiencing Depression/ Anxiety described like this:

"I think the biggest thing is my expectations I put on myself and what family members expect of me. I feel like I let them down or myself down because I can't do things like I use to. Some family members have termed me as lazy, which hurts."

She says the worst thing about CHF is:

"SOB and energy. Also, it's misunderstood by even doctor. I was going back and forth for about a year knowing something was wrong but no one could find out what/why."

This is the story she wanted to share:

I want to make this long story as short as possible because I'd fear I'd bore you with all the details. LOL!! However, I think it takes most of my almost 59 years to do so—at least most of it. What led to what is still the 64-thousand-dollar question because we don't know. All I remember from childhood is that I was born with an ASD (Atrial septal defect). I found out not long ago from one of my sisters that my parents knew about this when I was a baby but I didn't remember finding anything out about it until I was about 15 or 16. I was always kind of slow at school as far as participating in sports or Physical Ed etc. I was behind and was short of breath a lot of times, but not asthma. When I was about 15 my family doctor decided that we should see a cardiologist who ran some more tests and did a heart catheterization it was determined then that I had a hole in my heart or at least that's when I found out. Who knows they may have known about it before?? They told me at that time it wasn't really causing any issues that fixing it may or may not help the symptoms I was having and it was a pure choice whether or not to do open heart surgery to repair it. (That was in the 1970's and Open-heart surgery was the only way to fix it at that time. The newer technology with the patches that could be inserted via catheter hadn't even been developed yet). My parents were going thru other issues at the time so we decided to put it on hold for a while. Fast forward about 9-10 years later I was ready to get married and start a family. During a required physical for a California marriage license the subject came up again and at this point they thought it was imperative that if I were to have a family we needed to get this thing fixed. Although, non-invasive patches were successfully being used because my hole was so large and the location they thought it best to do open heart surgery and repair it that way. They did and it turned out very successful with a good recovery. I still had an enlarged heart but the problem was fixed. As it turned out, I was never able to have children of my own due to other issues I had but it had nothing to do with my heart. I still had issues with shortness of breath and fatigue in the next twenty, twenty-five years that followed but no one could figure it out. I did have occasions where I had some different surgeries and had some really weird funky heart beats. One particular occasion was in 2010 when I had my gallbladder removed. The anesthesiologist had noticed a really funky rhythm and wanted me to stay an extra couple of days in the hospital so they could monitor me and figure out what was going on. Then my surgeon came in a few minutes later and said nope it was just my heart for some reason and to let me go. I'd really wished they'd kept me because I knew at that time something wasn't right but we still couldn't figure it out. I'd been noticing my heart would race and my legs would occasionally swell but mostly they just blamed it on weight and lack of activity. In January of 2013, I had a fall on some ice and bummed up my knee so I started Physical Therapy to help strengthen it. I was then where I started having more issues of lightheadedness, heart racing way fast etc. They about called the ambulance on me during one of my PT sessions because my heart rate was up so high but it came down to a reasonable level when I stopped but they told me not to come back until I'd seen a doctor. It took a few more months before they finally diagnosed me with AFIB and almost a year before the Sick Sinus was diagnosed. Basically, my heart would go between fast and slow rates and rhythms. An Echo as far as I knew didn't show any heart damage, failure or abnormalities except for the AFIB, and SVT. Medications helped but made me feel like a zombie, so summer of 2013 I underwent an Ablation to try put a stop to the AFIB. Seemed to help somewhat but still had break thru AFIB. Because of the patch my EP couldn't get to the right side of the heart where he thought some of the problems existed, so he put me on a different rhythm medicine, which didn't have the zombie side effects the Metoprolol had. In early 2014, I was at work when from about my waist up I went numb and tingly which earned me my first ambulance ride. It was only a couple of blocks from my work to the hospital, but none the less, I took my very first ride. (Since then it's only been repeated once and hopefully will be no more LOL.) They couldn't really find anything wrong and diagnosed me with vertigo which I'd never had before and parenthesis. This actually earned me a monitor for a month and found out my heart rate sank every time I came out of AFIB, and I had pauses so I got a pacemaker. Which seemed to help. I was actually doing really well for a while then just when I thought I was over this, I started getting lightheaded and dizzy once again. Yep break thru AFIB yet again. This time my EP really did think it was an issue with the right side of my heart that he couldn't Ablate because of the patch. They'd tried me on a different medicine and within a couple of days they found out that there was no way that I could take it—especially with my PM or it could kill me—too bad because I actually thought I was beginning to feel better. It was then decided that they would need to go in and do another open-heart Maze procedure. They could burn the problem areas on the right side of my heart and hopefully correct the issue. So, on St. Patrick's day of 2015, I underwent a 2nd open heart surgery. I'm not sure all what they accomplished the hope was to put a stop to the AFIB, unfortunately I'm still on meds to this day. Although there was a time that I was completely off all of my medications for about 4 months! That was wonderful and I was so thankful. I also felt terrific! However, it was short lived once again. I had developed some issues with my eyesight and was referred to a specialist. They initially thought I had an issue with the cornea of my eye but while I did somewhat the bigger issue was cataracts! WHAT?? You've got to be kidding me I was only 56! On the first attempt with my first eye to have it removed, my heart went crazy! They had to stop the procedure and I had my second ambulance ride! They thought at that point I was having a PM issue because my heart was beating so weird.

So, I instead of having cataract surgery sat in the ER all day. Well I'm not sure what happened after that. They made some adjustments on my pacemaker—although it wasn't malfunctioning they changed some of the settings. Why to this day I do not know why or what or even what the reasoning behind it was, but from that point on I was in trouble and started to decline health wise still no one (doctors) was ready to blame it on the settings change or my heart, although I knew deep inside that something was done to the settings that screwed me up. For the next couple of years, my shortness of breath got worse, I was more tired I felt like crap. An easy 40-hour week at work became 4 days then down to 3. I just couldn't work anymore than that and still come home and have family to take care of. I was exhausted! My family was suffering and I was at wits end. I was beginning to think I was the one that was crazy! I was actually laid off in early 2016 due to my job being seasonal and it was a blessing in disguise because I was trying to also get ready for my daughter's wedding and I just couldn't do it. Meanwhile, I'd been bounced around between my EP and my PCP no it's not your heart, yes, it is your heart etc. my PCP finally thought it might be asthma and started aggressive treatment for that which did nothing. My legs continued to swell most of the time. I found the colder months weren't as bad. No one had suggested it was time to see a regular cardiologist. I had trusted my EP and when someone did mention that maybe I should —it never crossed my mind. I didn't fully understand the difference between an EP and a regular cardiologist. When my initial echo was done in 2013 I was referred to an EP. So never did it cross my mind that I needed a regular cardiologist. Hindsight if I had, things might have been a little different I'm wondering. Who knows?? Thanksgiving Day of 2016 I think was a turning point. (I'd known about CHF for a while—not that I knew I had it but watched both my uncle and grandmother deal with it, albeit years ago but I've had family members with it. I noticed my own symptoms and although they were beginning to reach familiar territory, I was refusing to admit that it might be after all the doctors didn't give me any indication that it even could be. I'm just a layman and know nothing but I do know my own body and I knew something was wrong. My daughter had heard about a Thanksgiving gourmet buffet up at a local ski resort only about a 45-minute drive from where we live. We were excited to go but once I got up there (I live at an altitude of about 4200 feet. The dinner was at about 7000 feet.) I knew I was in trouble! My SOB became major SOB and I was uncomfortable! My chest was hurting and I couldn't catch my breath! I made it thru dinner because I didn't want to ruin it for anyone, however I was very anxious to get off the mountain. I thought as soon as I got back to lower ground I would feel better. Unfortunately, I was still miserable after about an hour and I called the 24-hr. nurse line for advice. It was advised that I go straight to the ER. She asked if I needed an ambulance and I said no I'd have my husband take me. It wasn't that far away. Only about a 4 or 5-minute drive. Less than a couple of miles. So, we spent the rest of the evening in the ER. Yes, I was in active CHF! Finally, someone admitted it!! Then the big decision were they going to admit me or not. They weren't sure, however in the end because they felt that I'd been dealing with this for a while now. Hey wait a minute, this was the first time that anyone had actually told me I had CHF! But oh well!! They decided to send me home with a big IV dose of Lasix before I left. Ok wait a minute I was very glad I didn't have to stay —who wants to stay right??!! But come on—CHF?? Really?? At least now I knew what I was dealing with and why I'd been feeling like crap for so long. Finally, an answer! Oh, it gets better! I go back to my EP for follow up and meantime the surgeon is wanting to see me again for the follow up from the surgery he did the previous year—they like PM readings to check for the AFIB etc. and low and behold when they do the PM reading this time they actually find the weird setting that was changed the year before!! All along I knew something was screwed! They still didn't want to admit that was what was causing my issues and it may not have been because even when they set it back I didn't notice much improvement. But at least now we know what we're dealing with. I still didn't really have a plan on how to tackle this and still wasn't seeing a regular cardiologist just my EP. A new year (2017) begins and because my husband's employer changes insurance companies, I have to change doctors and hospitals if I want to stay within the network. No real plan for the CHF but before the year changed I did get a new Echo—which to this day don't know the report other than it did show signs of CHF. Probably diastolic since that's what the Echo 8 months later showed. I started going to a new EP who was not much help for the heart failure portion of it. My AFIB is almost nil, PM performing great follow up in 6 months. I'm not really doing any better so another echo is ordered and Pulmonary Function Tests (PFT's) were ordered. By mid-August, I'm struggling!! I'm trying to work part time as a cashier. I can't half breathe, my legs are like balloons and I can't walk 10 ft without literally panting like a dog. I stopped at a nearby 7-11 to get something for my son or granddaughter and I can barely get out of the car. In the car next to me was a nurse who literally wanted to take me up to the ER or call an ambulance, which the Fire department was just across the street. Of course, I refused saying I had testing the next day which I did. And once again I spent the afternoon in the ER! This time I really was almost admitted but not because of CHF but because they thought I had a blood clot. Fortunately, I didn't and once again CHF. But this time I'm finally getting somewhere by the end of that month I'd seen a heart failure doctor and was actually getting somewhere. Finally, someone is getting it and starting to LISTEN!! I'm sent for a Catheterization and was told to not work anymore that I had PH (Pulmonary hypertension) and diastolic heart failure. HELLO??!! Why in the heck did it take so LONG for someone to FINALLY figure it out??!! Now I'm finally getting treatment. Looking back, I wonder if some of the signs were there and if they'd been recognized if they could have been treated and I may have avoided the open-heart surgery in 2015?? Probably not. Basically, because I probably didn't have the issues back then. Yes, I had the AFIB but it wasn't until later after the Ablation in 2013 and Cox Maze in 2015 that I REALLY started having problems. We still don't know if any of this prior stuff is related or not. In January I saw a PH specialist who I've been working with for several months as we try to figure all of this out. I think I'm pretty much done with him though after a few more tests. I'm still lightheaded and dizzy at times but four of the meds I take can also cause that as well as the heart failure itself. There was a ton of scarring found when I had my second open heart surgery in 2015 and they are not sure if that's playing any kind of a role in how my heart is functioning or not. Since there was a lot of scarring then, I'm probably dealing with a lot now which might be causing my heart to be stiff. It was found that I do have stiff left atrial syndrome which they're saying is caused by right sided heart failure. Not quite understanding it all. I guess the good news is my Ejection Fraction is preserved but since my Atrium is stiff and won't relax between contractions it can't fill properly. I'm still not getting the volume *of blood circulating that I should be. With the lightheadedness that I'm experiencing now, my PCP recommended that I see a PT who ran some testing on my eye tracking and balance. I had a VNG (Videonystagmography) with an audiologist and they've determined that I might have some CNS (Central Nervous System) issue so I'm waiting for brain MRI and neurology consult. As far as my heart failure itself it seems to be improving at least somewhat. I did do Cardiac Rehab for a while, however when summer started I had to stop because of scheduling conflicts with my daughter. (I take care of my grandson while she's working) The PH specialist increased my diuretics and is trying to more aggressively treat it. Four of the medicines I currently take can cause lightheadedness and or dizziness as well as the condition itself. So sometimes it seems I'm trading off one thing for another. After the Catheterization last September, they reduced my PM lower limit to 50 in hopes of giving my heart more time to fill. With the increased lightheadedness, I was curious if that what was causing the issues, since that's one of the reasons I got the PM to begin with. So, they've increased it back up to 60 —one trade off sometimes for another. Good news is my heart rate and BP are up where they were so low before—but sometimes I seem to be more short of breath but I could be anyway. Not really sure if it's really helping at this point.*

It seems right now the important thing is learning to find the balancing act between enough and too much fluids, salt etc. watching your weight and sticking to the low salt diet.

I'm still in the process of trying to get disability since my doctor last year told me after the catheterization not to work anymore. I've been denied twice already—for anyone in this boat DON'T GIVE UP—actually I think SS wants you to give up—that's why they deny you so many times."

Gerald   Mastic Beach, NY   (#32)

Gerald is a Caregiver in the CHF world for 2 years. (Caregivers were asked to respond about the patient they care for.)

The main symptoms they experience are explained as, *"fluid retention"*.

CHF has impacted their quality of life to some degree.

They are being treated with the following medications:

"Entresto, Eliquis, B6, iron, Pantoprazole, Duloxetine, Benadryl, Trazadone, aspirin, Levothyroxine, Atorvastatin, Amiodarone, Carvedilol, Furosemide, Spironolactone, Glimepiride."

They are <u>not</u> experiencing Depression/ Anxiety.

They say the worst thing about CHF is:

"Breathing difficulties and weak legs."

This is the story they wanted to share:

" Didn't feel any symptoms of the first heart attack, slight nausea and weakness. Drove car and loaded and unloaded trailer. Later just felt weakness and vomiting. Was told if I didn't go straight to hospital she was calling an ambulance. Received 5 stents. Then a second heart attack when they were diagnosed with CHF. Waiting in car to bring boys home from

work. Felt tightness then couldn't get my breath in or out. Ambulance called. Received 7 stents. Had a third heart attack, felt pain and pressure. Forth heart attack legs were swollen had 5xCABG. Mitral valve repair. After coding at nurse's station their heart was pumped till entered CABG surgery. Fifth heat attack on operating table. Wore life vest for 4 months. Legs were swollen. Defibrillator was implanted."

Thanks for sharing this story.

Jeffrey M.   Ord, NB   (#33)

Jeffrey is a more experienced member in the CHF world and has had it for 20 years.

The main symptoms he experiences are explained this way:

"Pain, Edema, VTAC, VFIB and AFIB."

CHF has <u>not</u> impacted his quality of life very much.

Jeffrey said he is being treated with, "a *lot of medications*".

He is experiencing Depression/ Anxiety described like this:

"Harder to work."

He says the worst thing about CHF is:

"Dealing with insurance companies, and the medical system in general."

This is the story he wanted to share:

"Work hard, play hard. Guess I played too hard."

Name Withheld   *Calverton, NY*   *(#34)*

This member is very new to the CHF world and has been involved for less than a year.

The symptoms they experience are explained this way:

"ZERO, I am still not convinced I have it, despite the low EF rating on numerous tests.

CHF has impacted their quality of life explained this way:

"So far it is a horrible experience of doctors and referrals who seem to only care about one thing, what can we get the insurance to cover."

They are being treated with the following medications:

"Plavix, Lisinopril, Metoprolol and Atorvastatin."

They experiencing Depression/ Anxiety described like this:

"Tons of anxiety. I don't understand why they keep pushing me to get a defibrillator when I'm told it will only ever activate in 10 percent of people, will do nothing for quality of life and has risks as well as needing battery changes forever. I don't qualify for a pacemaker which seems like something I could go for, but just the defibrillator? I am disheartened that most info online seems to be from the makers of the devices and a Netflix documentary called "the bleeding edge" makes me even more leery of this.

I am not convinced these medications are doing anything positive for me. I think it is very difficult to trust doctors in the American for profit medical system."

They say the worst thing about CHF is:

"Trying to find information that is not slanted by drug or device makers."

No Life story was shared!

Virginia B.   Minot, ND (#35)

Virginia is another newer member in the CHF world and has been with us for 3 months.

The main symptoms she experiences are explained this way:

"Severe Edema, inability to take satisfying breaths, shortness of breath, heaviness in chest, extreme fatigue and dizziness"

CHF has impacted her quality of life described like this:

"Unable to complete simple tasks, fatigue keeps me in bed a lot, can't work."

Virginia is being treated with medications:

"Blood pressure, Carvedilol, Lasix and potassium supplement"

She is experiencing Depression/ Anxiety described like this:

"I struggled with depression and anxiety before but it is exacerbated now. It's hard to find purpose in my days. I'm so limited and my anxiety gets very bad over self-doubts with taking care of my family."

She says the worst thing about CHF is:

"Not being able to just live my life."

This is the story she wanted to share:

"I was 38 and over the course of six months my body just seem to rebel against me. I work a job where I stand all day but only part time and it got to the point where slowly I lost all of my stamina. I never imagined that there was something more going on. It went from extreme fatigue to severe swelling in my legs and ankles to shortness of breath and finally to completely not being able to function in my daily life. I couldn't walk more than 10 feet without having to rest and everything winded me and made me feel so sick. I was convinced it was something completely different when I finally dragged myself to the ER. They were looking for blood clots in my lungs when they did a chest CT and then they discovered a massive amount of fluid around my heart. It has been a very long journey and I'm only at the beginning. I couldn't do it without the love and support of my family and my church. I have been very blessed to be surrounded by people who are willing to help. I still feel trapped and angry some days but most days I just try to take it an hour at a time and not focus too much on the future. I have and Ejection Fraction of 20%. I'll have another echo done in 3 months and see if it has improved. They believe it was caused by a virus and I have no heart disease or blockages. This is the hardest thing I have ever done."

Thanks for sharing this information.

Shirley C.   Panama City, FL(#36)

Shirley has been in the CHF world for 4 years.

The main symptoms she experiences are explained this way:

"Weight gain, Edema, memory loss, dizziness, pain. I am short of breath much of the time. I have swelling in my legs. I have problems with memory loss. At times my blood pressure drops and I get dizzy. I have back pains and sometimes chest pains. I also have acid indigestion quite a bit."

CHF has impacted her quality of life described like this:

"I can't do many of the things I used to. I was a math tutor online and now I struggle to remember many of the formulas and methods. I also struggle to do my normal things around the house or to go to festivals or events where walking is involved."

Shirley is being treated with medications:

"Lasix, Carvedilol, and Entresto. I also take Famotidine and a regular aspirin daily at the direction of my doctor."

She is experiencing Depression/ Anxiety described like this:

"I don't think I have anxiety or depression, but I do stress more easily since being diagnosed."

She says the worst thing about CHF is:

"The memory loss and having to monitor sodium intake and fluid intake so closely. Also not being able to do things I used to do with the family."

This is the story she wanted to share:

"I was having trouble breathing and had a bad cough for several months. My ankles were also very swollen but I thought it was a chest cold and kept trying to ease the symptoms by taking OTC meds and sleeping sitting up. Finally, it got so bad I couldn't breathe even just sitting and went to the ER. I was diagnosed with CHF with an EF less than 10%. Within days I had an ICD implanted and had dropped about 15 lbs. of fluid. I was sent home with the instructions to put down the salt shaker to limit sodium to 1500 mg per day along with potassium, Spironolactone, Carvedilol, Lisinopril, Furosemide, Famotidine, and baby aspirin as my meds. I soon discovered that putting the salt shaker down was just a fraction of the sodium in our diets and did a lot of research and found that I had to completely change my diet to reduce my sodium intake. I was feeling tingling in my fingers and face and when I went for my first blood test after a few weeks, I was rushed to the hospital with a dangerous level of potassium. My kidneys were not functioning as they should. After about 2 weeks in the hospital my potassium was back to normal almost and the doctor discontinued the Spironolactone and the potassium. They monitored my kidneys and they are functioning almost at a normal level once again. My EF went up to about 25% after 2 years and then dropped back to 20%. I was then switched to Entresto instead of Lisinopril. I am due for an echo next month and I am hoping for good news although I continue to be short of breath and experience swelling in spite of monitoring my sodium intake and faithfully taking the meds. I get frustrated with my inability to do normal everyday things but I am thankful to be alive and hopefully will improve and be able to live with CHF for quite a while."

Jim B.   *Winchester, VA   (#37)*

Jim has been in the CHF world for 4 1/2 years.

The main symptoms he experiences are explained this way:

"Weight gain, Edema, memory loss, dizziness, pain and shortness of breath."

CHF has impacted his quality of life described like this:

"I still work full time but need a lot of rest."

Jim is being treated with medications:

"Coreg, Lipitor, Plavix, Losartan, Lasix and a baby aspirin."

He is experiencing Depression/ Anxiety described like this:

"Anxiety, panic attacks and lack sleep."

He says the worst thing about CHF is:

"People think I am completely recovered and should be fine."

This is the story he wanted to share:

"02/06/2014 I had a massive heart attack and cardiac arrest. I was in a coma for 6 days. I got 4 stents and a pacemaker as soon as I woke from the coma, went thru cardiac rehabilitation and was back to work 8 weeks later. I have since had 2 stents collapse and have to be repaired, and had a bout of Sepsis, 9 days in hospital. I am fighting every day, taking my meds and going to the gym 3 days a week to live my best life."

Thanks for sharing this information.

Megan   Denver, CO(#38)

Megan is pretty new to the CHF world and has had it 6 months.

The main symptoms she experiences are explained this way:

"Before treatment, dizziness, shortness of breath and Edema."

CHF has impacted her quality of life described like this:

"Made me change my lifestyle. Changed eating habits and I stopped taking things for granted."

Megan is being treated with medications:

"Lisinopril and Coreg."

She is <u>not</u> experiencing Depression/ Anxiety.

She says the worst thing about CHF is:

"Feeling different."

She did not choose to share a story.

Bob H.   *London, Ontario, Canada*   (#39)

Bob has been in the CHF world for only 1 year.

The main symptoms he experiences are explained this way:

"I get mental fog and/or memory loss. Actually, have lost weight due to diet change. I tend to overheat easily and find myself being weaker slowly over time. What used to be a piece of cake now requires rest. I also deal with fatigue and if my anxiety increases my heart rate goes with it."

CHF has impacted his quality of life described like this:

"I've had to stop working. Have to stay indoors more because of the heat. Stress on the family in regards to the news and understanding my CHF. But I am changing my routines, my diet, etc. I have found that I have been feeling better more days than not. My EF is at 22%."

Bob is being treated with medications:

"Myriad of medications. I suffer spinal damage. So I take Gabapentin, Tylenol 4, Baclofen, Amitriptyline, Bupropion, Bisoprolol, Perindopril, Furosemide."

He is experiencing Depression/ Anxiety described like this:

"At first it was a deep depression, but as I settled down and took stock of it, I had to learn to deal with it. If I get caught up too much in the why me, I'll

never enjoy what I have. So, I have my bad days, moments and cries. But, I am always going to laugh, smile and enjoy those around me and those that are dear to my heart."

He says the worst thing about CHF is:

"The stigma. You get told you have CHF and the first thing you do is wonder if you're going to die soon. There's not a lot of down to earth helpful information. My diet was comprised of nothing but no food from a box or a can. I want to show people that it's never too late. But CHF is going to be with you, just wish there was better info to help us deal with the options."

This is the story he wanted to share:

"Pretty easy. I had been suffering from a cough for quite a while and my doctor told me it could just be a left over from the cold season and prescribed me puffers. Now the puffers did help but, I still had the cough. Girlfriend bugs me to go the urgent care center. It was Easter and I succumbed to her urging. They did the blood work, the x-ray, the look down your throat and the breath in breath out stuff. But for a fluke the doctor decided to put me on an EKG monitor to see what was happening there. He had discovered that it showed I had left bundle branch blocked. Knowing nothing about it I was kind of scared. He said I'm going to refer you to a Heart specialist just to make sure everything is going to be OK. Week later I see the Heart Doc and he said it looks like I have cardiomyopathy. He scheduled me for an echo and an MRI. Did the echo they called me back 3 days later. It shows that I had a significant EF% drop. I was at 22%. He said we're going to schedule you for an Angiogram. Go to the Angiogram have that sucker shoved up my wrist to my heart. After checking it all out he said "sorry nothing I can do. You have no plugged or collapsed arteries. I will refer you to the heart failure clinic". Then he left *without waiting to answer any questions I may have had. So, faced with this knowledge needless to say I was completely devastated. No one wants to be told your dying, but at least stay for some questions. It was a week after that, when I see my GP and she gave me the results. This happened all within 3 weeks from start to finish. And to think it all started with just a cough."*

Thanks for sharing this information.

Allison S.   *Platte, SD*   (#40)

Allison has been in the CHF world for only 5 years.

The main symptoms she experiences are explained this way:

"Muscle loss, sleepless nights, acid reflux, tiredness when walking, skin rashes, cold hands and feet"

CHF has impacted her quality of life described like this:

"Hard to keep up with my 9-yr. old. Getting used to not being able and afraid to go do certain things or adventures by myself because I run out of "spoons".

Allison is being treated with medications:

"5 different ones."

She did not respond on Depression/ Anxiety.

She says the worst thing about CHF is:

"Not being able to do things on my own."

This is the story she wanted to share:

"47 years old and I have CHF and Alpha-1 and Pulmonary hypertension."

Thanks for sharing this information.

Name Withheld Brookfield, WI   (#41)

This member has been in the CHF world for 6 years.

The main symptoms they experience are explained this way:

"Weight gain, Edema, memory loss, light headed, pain, shortness of breath, palpitations, nauseous, weak, tired and sometimes touchy."

CHF has impacted his quality of life described like this:

"Very limited on what I can do and can never predict when I will feel good enough to participate in life activities."

The member is being treated with medications:

"Losartan, Coreg and Wellbutrin."

They are experiencing Depression/ Anxiety described like this:

"Tired and temperamental."

They say the worst thing about CHF is:

"Wanting to do things and when I start I just can't do them. I hate having others having to carry my responsibilities. That is not what a partnership is. Feel guilty about not being a complete partner to my husband."

This is the story they wanted to share:

"I was not feeling well and wanted to get back into shape. I was going to school and could hardly carry my books to class. I went to the doctor for a physical. He did blood work for the physical, we met he said everything was fine and that I could start a physical activity program with no restrictions. I also was going to have my eyes lifted and that doctor wanted a physical also, only they also needed an EKG. (why my regular PCP did not want one I don't know) the nurse ran the EKG and ran into the doctor's office. I had a LBBB and the doctor then wanted an Echo and stress test. Fortunately, the Echo was done first because when it was time to do the stress test, they didn't want to do it because I was in agony. They looked at the echo and put me in the hospital for 3 days diagnosing me with CHF with EF 35%. Now remember my primary said that I was fine, when I went back for follow up with him, he said "Oh you are the patient that created the most excitement we had in this office in a long time." I was diagnosed with DCM idiopathic, and frequent PVCs, went to an EP had two ablations and the last one was so deep, I had a small heart attack. I have an ICD that has not gone off, but am now referred to advanced cardiac heart failure and going into more testing as very symptomatic even with EF of 37%."

Thanks for sharing this information.

Tea M.   *Gastonia, NC*   (#42)

Tea has been in the CHF world since diagnosed in March 2018.

The main symptoms she experiences are explained this way:

"My mind goes blank a lot. My bones ache. I can gain 5 lbs. of fluid following fluid and sodium restrictions. My blood pressure stays very low so I'm dizzy often. My endurance is almost nonexistent."

CHF has impacted her quality of life described like this:

"My quality of life is what I'm trying to improve right now by doing cardiac rehab. I have anxiety but am pushing forward to be able to attend events with my children who are 15, 13, 10, and 8 still at home. I'm grateful for everyday I'm blessed to see. My goal is to live to watch my baby girl graduate. I'm stubborn and have a strong will to live. When I was hospitalized for this the doctors didn't think I would live 3 days. Upon discharge with a CRT-D implanted, I gained 110 lbs. of fluid for which I was readmitted for 1 month of IV Lasix to remove the fluid. I was told then that I'm stage 4 and had swelling due to CHF. They also said I have every cardiac disease known to man. My heart is heavily damaged with lots of blockages. Surgery won't help me unless I get a transplant. My heart is paced at 70 and my device and meds help my weak heartbeat."

Tea is being treated with medications:

"Insulin, Lasix, potassium, Carvedilol, Lisinopril, Amiodarone and Clopidogrel."

She is experiencing Depression/ Anxiety described like this:

"Both. I fight to be positive and relaxed. I know I have a CRT-D but worry about my heart giving out."

She says the worst thing about CHF is:

"Being stuck in a defective body wanting to do things like before. Once I was able to hold down 2 jobs now I can't work at all."

This is the story she wanted to share:

"I'm trying to fight my way back to pre-CHF level. I have more bad days than good right now. I lost both breasts, my ovaries, and my hair, eyelashes and eyebrows to breast cancer and the strong chemo damaged my heart along with diabetes and high blood pressure. Teach your children to eat right. Leave fast food alone."

Thanks for sharing this story.

Debbie F.   *Philadelphia, PA*   *(#43)*

Debbie has had CHF for 9 months and was actually diagnosed 6 months ago.

The main symptoms she experiences are explained this way:

"Massive weight gain, Edema, coughing, congestion and loss of breath."

CHF has impacted her quality of life described like this:

"Changed my way of life for the better, along with my family. We exercise, make healthy food decisions, quit smoking, relax more to minimize stress."

Debbie is being treated with medications:

"Furosemide (Lasix), Lisinopril and Baby Aspirin."

She is experiencing Depression/ Anxiety described like this:

"Anxiety when going out to dinner because I know my food choices are limited and don't want people feeling sorry for me. Since being diagnosed, I've gone into a funk two times, but realized both times that I am alive and have loved ones who support me. The support usually snaps me out of it."

She says the worst thing about CHF is:

"Knowing that I am not invincible. Knowing that at any time I can drop dead. Knowing that my life has changed and I can either deal or die.."

This is the story she wanted to share:

"After suffering with what I thought was bronchitis, I finally went to cardiologist who immediately put me in the hospital for 7 days. Over the course of that week, I had two cardiac Catheterizations, lost almost 30 lbs. of fluid and stopped breathing three times. Since then, I've learned to love my doctors, follow their orders, lost now almost 50 lbs., made major life style changes and have made sure that my family understands the need to change their lives. I am currently being evaluated for an ICD and or transplant. My EF has gone from 11% to 20%. I consider myself very lucky because according to my cardiologist, I was 2-3 weeks away from having a major heart attack when I was first seen by him. The worst thing to know is that my CHF is still unknown, as to the cause."

Thanks for sharing this story.

Jocelyn V.   Gordonsville, VA (#44)

Jocelyn has is pretty experienced in the CHF world having it for 13 years.

The main symptoms she experiences are explained this way:

"Shortness of breath, fluid retention, swelling, fatigue, weight gain and memory loss."

CHF has impacted her quality of life described like this:

"I am so fatigued that I sleep 15 hours a day which includes a 2 hour nap. It makes it difficult to walk distances or climb stairs due to shortness of breath. Some nights I can't breathe well so I have to sleep in a recliner. I feel like a water balloon!"

Jocelyn is being treated with medications:

"Lasix, Metoprolol, Lisinopril, Spironolactone, Nitroglycerin, Ranexa, Effient and Crestor."

She is not experiencing Depression/ Anxiety but describes it like this:

"I 'm not depressed or anxious but I am lonely and bored."

She says the worst thing about CHF is:

"When it first kicked in on the operating table my lungs filled with fluid and I couldn't breathe. It was scary and felt like I was drowning. I pray I never feel that bad again!"

This is her CHF story shared via e-mail:

"Started with rheumatoid arthritis at age 24 but was active - avid golfer. Taught elementary schools for 28 years when one day, at age 49, had a T.I.A with temporary vision loss. Sent to UVA hospital where CTA of brain and carotid arteries showed a rare disease of my arteries called FMD or Fibromuscular Dysplasia, 2 stents implanted in carotid arteries-one dissected, the other had an aneurysm. Sudden very high BP, kidney arteries ballooned open - FMD here also. Two months later, I had 2 heart attacks 3 days apart at Christmas time. Both with crushing chest pain, nausea, sweating and incredible fatigue that made me so weak I couldn't talk. Arrived in ER with BP 90/0 in cardiogenic shock and coronary artery 100% stenosed and dissected! Two stents implanted awoke to not being able to breathe, CHF started. ER cardiologists said they had never seen anyone survive a heart attack as bad as mine, so my cardiologist nicknamed me Miracle Girl. Spent 3 weeks in ICCU and 1 week in step down then regular heart floor. I get chest pain frequently from a lot of permanent damage if I exert myself doing simple things. Frequently, I have to use my power wheelchair from severe CHF besides. But, I thank God every day that I am still alive. He had a plan and I am just his paint brush."

Thanks for sharing this information.

Sheila M.   Philadelphia, PA   (#45)

Sheila has been in the CHF world for 5 years.

The main symptoms she experiences are explained this way:

"Weight gain, Edema, dizziness, chest pain, high blood pressure, heart palpitations and heart murmur."

CHF has impacted her quality of life described like this:

"I cannot do the things I used to do. My quality of life is bad I am stuck in the house."

Sheila is being treated with medications:

"Torsemide, Lisinopril, Coreg, and potassium and two more blood pressure pills."

She is experiencing Depression/ Anxiety described like this:

"Yes, depression and anxiety. I am scared to sleep because I don't want to die in my sleep and I'm sad because I can't do the things I used to do and I can't really enjoy life."

She says the worst thing about CHF is:

"Not being able to breathe and can't sleep."

This is the story she wanted to share:

"I was diagnosed in 2013 after years of walking and being out of breath and having high blood pressure. I went to the ER and they told me, but I didn't take it seriously. I was put on water pills but was rarely taking them. I also was still having blood pressure problems and eating whatever but never took it serious till I almost died. I rode from California to Georgia and was swollen up big. I was admitted in the hospital May 2017 for a week where I had test and heart failure classes. I haven't slept flat in a bed since 2006 and it sucks."

Thanks for sharing this story.

Darlene B.   Florence, SC   (#46)

Darlene has been in the CHF world for 6 years.

The main symptoms she experiences are explained this way:

"Weight gain, wheezing and exhaustion (all the time)."

CHF has impacted her quality of life described like this:

"Because of another ailment, my quality of life had been poor for some time. The beta blocker has only made it worse."

Darlene is being treated with medications but says:

"The list is ridiculously long."

She is experiencing Depression/ Anxiety described like this:

"At first, I was anxious all the time. Since stopping Carvedilol, the depression and anxiety is almost nonexistent."

She says the worst thing about CHF is:

"Choosing what I am able to eat."

This is the story she wanted to share:

"My CHF hit about 6-7 weeks after a heart attack. That night is emblazoned in my mind. I was in and out of it in the ambulance. I remember hearing the paramedic calling in my vitals on the way to the hospital. Blood pressure was 240/140. When I got the ER and was rolled into the exam room, there was a respiratory therapist there with a ventilator waiting on me. I was close to death. About 18 months after that, the same cardiologist in the ER was also the one who did my sister's heart cath. He shook my brother-in-law's hand and they introduced themselves. He looked at me and said, "I know who you are". I'm thankful and blessed to be alive."

Thanks for sharing this story.

Cindi L.   Hillsboro, MO   (#47)

Cindi is new to the CHF world and has had it since Dec 25, 2017.

The main symptoms she experiences are explained this way:

> *"Weak, memory lost, leg pain gained over 50lbs in 7 months and out of breath to name a few."*

CHF has impacted her quality of life described like this:

> *"I have no life can't do anything really. Quality is not good. Just got a CRT-D, 4 weeks ago hoping it changes soon but, no change yet."*

Cindi is being treated with medications but says:

> *"Cholesterol, dietetics, blood pressure, they seem to change every Doctor visit."*

She is experiencing Depression/ Anxiety described like this:

> *"Depression and the will to live because it changed my whole life. Can't work, can't take care of myself. Went from working 14 hours a day 7 days a week to can't hardly walk from the couch to the bathroom. It gets to me."*

She says the worst thing about CHF is:

"No life and pain and no breath."

This is the story she wanted to share:
"Woke up on Christmas Eve went down to my basement to get Christmas presents to go to my daughter's house and I could not get up the steps. I was so out of breath it took me 7 breaks to get to the top of the landing. I wasn't sick at all, I concluded that I must have pneumonia. Went to my daughter's celebrated Christmas, but bailed out early. On my way home I thought maybe I'll stop at the emergency room and get some antibiotics because it was the first time I had been off work three good days in a row for the holidays. I thought I can take the antibiotics rest up and I'll be fine. Got to the emergency room they took blood, EKG and then they took an Echo that's when I found out my heart EF was only at 13%. Then my nightmare started. I never have felt good since that day. My local hospital had a cardiologist on staff, so I started seeing him he tried all kinds of different medications kept me in the hospital on and off for the next 6 months (7 times) until I got another Echocardiogram that showed in 6 months of taking all the medicine, I had no change in my EF which was no good. He wanted to air lift me to St Louis Barnes Hospital and have a LVAD device put in, which scared me to death. He felt like it was necessary because my kidneys were starting to shut down. I beg for another day and another test on my kidneys, thank goodness I did my kidneys seem to settle down so there was no giant rush on getting the LVAD device. That was one of my biggest fears because I had been on an IV where I had to carry a bag around for months and months and it was horrible on the quality of my life. An LVAD you have to carry around an external battery so I was freaking out that for the rest of my life I would have some cord attached to me. Showers would be very difficult no swimming but I would be alive. The next 30 days I fought about the LVAD and decided I was not going to get it. Nothing seemed to be helping me in my disease, why would I go through all of that. My local cardiologist referred me to a cardiologist in Barnes Hospital, St Louis letting me know that they were the best in the world that I would be in great hands Went to meet my new cardiologist and heart transplant team they put me in the hospital and redid every test that I ever had since I had been diagnosed. They wanted to make their

own opinion and no one else's. They put me in the ICU and started testing me for a week after all tests were complete they concluded that I should get a CRT-D, which has all of batteries internally so I would not have to carry anything outside my body, everything would be inside so I was very happy about that. If in 6 months if no change, I will get on the heart transplant list. This disease is very hard on a person I don't have any type of life or social interaction. They talk about cardio rehabilitation which is a joke when you can't even walk to the bathroom without being worn out. You are dependent one hundred percent on other people. I feel my next step is to look for some kind of Assistant Living Facility."

Thanks for sharing this story.

Cordelia M.   *Victorville, CA*   (#48)

Cordelia has been in the CHF world for 6 years.

The main symptoms she experiences are explained this way:

"I have a lot of memory loss, swelling feet ankles and stomach, shortness of breath, a feeling of hopelessness. Dizziness, my weight goes up and down depends on if I'm retaining fluids."

CHF has impacted her quality of life described like this:

"I've lost a lot of friends and relationships because people think I'm faking. I can't do things without getting tired I have to pass up many opportunities because I get weak, Jobs etc. I feel old when I'm still kind of young."

Cordelia is being treated with medications described as:

"Coreg, Multaq, Lasix, Eliquis, Adempas, Entresto and much, much more."

She is experiencing Depression/ Anxiety described like this:

"Depression and feeling lost."

She says the worst thing about CHF is:

"The unknown. One day you can be feeling well and then you have a setback."

This is the story she wanted to share:

"I used to take care of my mom who died of Heart failure. One day I began to feel just like I saw how she felt, I was only 43. I went to the doctor, I told him I couldn't breathe he look at my shoes and said nice shoes. I said Doctor, I really can't breathe he finally gave me a chest x-ray and found out I was full of fluids. I stayed in the hospital for a week. After that every 2 months I was in hospital. I lost my jobs and struggled to even get dressed. Even when I applied for disability the Judged looked me and said, you don't look sick. He too thought I was faking because my outside didn't look like my inside. I felt sad and alone. I even thought suicide would be better. Being a care giver then a patient broke me down. Out of 6 sisters why me, I would think. I felt empty and alone. No good for anyone. My husband didn't care, my friends who I thought would be there were gone, only a small few had stayed. I couldn't breathe, Heart function 15%, when I first found out. I could walk but a couple of feet at first. I ended up with AFIB, chronic kidney disease and pulmonary Hypertension all stemming from my heart failure. But, I had a fight in me that I myself could understand. I was determined to live and not die. With the help of my heart doctor. I begin to change my eating habits and forcing myself to walk. I cut down on my fluids to only 32 oz. a day. CHF was not going to win, I'm going to win. Not to long ago I got a pacemaker /ICD and practice relaxing, for me dreaming about the ocean and the sun set on the waters. I saw myself walking further. Even When I laid in a hospital Bed, I knew it wouldn't be for long. I began to speak positive to myself even though my mind was trying to tell me something else. Now My Heart function is 55%, I have come a long way . There are still bad days, but I allow myself to rest on those days and I look forward to better days, because I want to dance, live, love and enjoy life. I want to appreciate things that most don't even think about, taking a big breath and breathing. Walking and putting on my *cloths, as long as I can. I can't complain. CHF, I'M GOING TO FIGHT UNTIL I CAN'T...."*

_____

Thanks for sharing this story.

Name Withheld Cherry Hill, NJ (#49)

This member has been in the CHF world for 5 years.

The main symptoms they experience are explained this way:

"Coughing. shortness of breath, feeling like I'm choking on my own sputum."

CHF has impacted their quality of life described like this:

"I was in a competitive nursing program and halfway I had quit going because I felt like it was too much for my heart to physically handle and mentally the stress wasn't good for me either. Prior to getting the ICD implanted, my quality of life was going down fast. I guess because I am so young I thought I could be invincible. After the ICD, it gave me the motivation to have a better quality of life not only because the ICD gave me a sense of peace, but also having one implanted is a wakeup call that at any moment my heart could stop, so I need to get my act together."

They are being treated with medications explained as:

"Digoxin, Furosemide, potassium, Spironolactone, Entresto and Metoprolol."

They are experiencing Depression/ Anxiety described like this:

"Depression definitely. I don't want to go before my mom passes away. Her mom, dad and sister all have passed away within 5 years of each other and I don't want to put that on her. Also, just feeling like no one understand what I'm going through and chalk it down to oh have her sit down for a minute and not understanding this isn't just a take a break situation. This is daily for me. Just as an example."

They say the worst thing about CHF is:

"Not being able to breath."

This is the story they wanted to share:

"Freshman year in college. I've been having this on and off again cough since Oct of 2012. It seemed to get worst as the winter progressed. I chalked it up to it just being winter. One night in Feb 2013 a group of friends and I went out to eat at a Chinese Restaurant (my favorite). Later that night I swore I was food poisoned because I was over the toilet coughing and vomiting the whole night. It came to a point where I slept in my apartment bathroom and now it was only clear liquids coming up. I decided that I was going to go to the ER later on in the afternoon. I get there and they told me I had a serve case of pneumonia and luckily, I came when I did. So, I was in there for 2 days receiving antibiotics. On the day I was supposed to be discharged my nurse noticed that my heart rate was 134 and I was sitting in bed. I have been in bed since I got there because I was drained from all the coughing and vomiting I was able to sleep. So, she monitored it for a couple hrs. and it kept fluctuating between 130-140. She noticed that wasn't right and asked the doctor to order an Echo. Surely enough, I had an Echo and the cardiologist on duty gave me the bad news. An older man came in (cardiologist) and sat down to describe to me what's going on. He stated that he has never seen someone this young (18, 19 in 4 more days) *having CHF with an EF of 25%. That literally tore me to pieces. I then was moved to the cardiac floor and stayed an additional 3 days. I eventually finished my freshman year and decided to move back home and attend a university closer to home. I found a new amazing cardiologist and started my treatment. Recently, at the end of 2017, I was going through this coughing phase and constantly feeling sluggish and tired and I couldn't breathe. I got hospitalized in March 2018 the first time since my initial hospitalization back in 2013 and again on a Friday in May of 2018. The ER I went to in May evaluated me and suggested I get transported to the hospital where my cardiologist works (PENN) and get an ICD placed. I got transported by ambulance to the other hospital and that following Tuesday I got my ICD implanted."*

Thanks for sharing this story.

Teresa P.   Mt. Holly, NC   (#50)

Teresa is very new to our CHF world since diagnosed in May 2018.

The main symptoms she experiences are explained this way:

"Weight gain, Edema and dizziness. Shortness of breath. It's easy for me to get tired."

CHF has impacted her quality of life described like this:

"I can't keep going and going without resting. It affects my anxiety levels. I stay home more now!"

Teresa is being treated with medications:

"No list was provided."

She is experiencing Depression/ Anxiety described like this:

"Anxiety! It makes my heart beat faster and I can't rest or function properly."

She says the worst thing about CHF is:

"Retaining fluid and being restricted to 64 oz. a day. I can't eat the food I love and getting tired easily."

This is the story she wanted to share:

"My journey just started so far I don't have much to report other than it was the scariest 4 days of my life. Not being able to breath is a scary thing."

Thanks for sharing this story.

Cathy S.   DeWitt, AR (#51)

Cathy has been in our CHF world for 7 years.

The main symptoms she experiences are explained this way:

"Weight gain , fatigued, shortness of breath, excess urination & heart palpitations."

CHF has impacted her quality of life described like this:

"I'm blessed every day I wake up . Blessed I'm get to see my daughters become adults."

Cathy is being treated with medications:

"Escitalopram, Hydroxyzine, Coq10, aspirin, Metoprolol and Simvastatin."

She is experiencing Depression/ Anxiety described like this:

"Anxiety - Afraid I'm going to have another heart attack. I go out to eat dinner occasionally. And I grocery shop. Besides that I'm at home cooking & cleaning."

She says the worst thing about CHF is:

"Gaining weight and being fatigued all the time. And shortness of breath."

This is the story she wanted to share:

"I had a heart attack in 2011. Anyway, I ended up getting a quadruple bypass. I died twice on the table . (That's what my ex-husband, daughters, & sister told me). Since my heart attack, I have gotten divorced. I'm blessing every moment with my daughters."

Thanks for sharing this story.

Carole C.   *Houston, TX*   *(#52)*

Carole is relatively new to our CHF world and has had it for 6 months.

The main symptoms she experiences are explained this way:

"Edema, shortness of breath and dizziness."

CHF has impacted her quality of life described like this:

"I get so tired so easy. Can't walk very far or very fast without having to rest or stop."

Carole is being treated with medications:

"Pravastatin, Lasix, potassium and Losartan."

She is experiencing Depression/ Anxiety described like this:

"Yes. Worrying about the future I also have MS and spine issues so that adds to depression and worries."

She says the worst thing about CHF is:

"For me, it's the shortness of breath Just can't keep up with everyone anymore."

This is the story she wanted to share:

"Hi I'm Carole. I have been a NICU nurse for 25 years. By the end of my shift my legs and feet would be huge tight and shiny with Edema. I had a chronic cough and was short of breath. Sometimes, my Doctor would tell me it's from being overweight and on my feet for a 12 hour shift. I was diagnosed 6 months ago after being so short of breath I could barely walk 50 feet without having to stop. That led to blood work, ECHO, Stress test and Cardiac Cath... 3 days in Hospital on IV Lasix... hello Diastolic CHF."

Thanks for sharing this story.

Paul S.   *Fort Wayne, IN*   *(#53)*

Paul is relatively new to our CHF world and has had it for 4 months.

The main symptoms he experiences are explained this way:

"Shortness of breath, dizziness and coughing."

CHF has impacted his quality of life described like this:

"Early on it limited my hours at work and my ability to get around. I also had dizzy spells and would pass out."

Paul is being treated with medications:

"I was diagnosed with AFIB and CHF. In the beginning: Digoxin, Losartan, potassium, Metoprolol, Amiodarone, Liothyronine, Xarelto. This was for the first 8 weeks, now taking: Amiodarone and Xarelto."

He is not experiencing Depression/ Anxiety he described it like this:

"I am very lucky: No depression I was very irritated and quick to snap in the beginning. Much less now. Drastic changes in diet. Lost 49 pounds so far. Just finishing up 24 sessions at Cardiac Rehab and I'm back on my road bike."

He says the worst thing about CHF is:

"Not knowing what is going on and if I will suddenly developed the more debilitating symptoms."

This is the story he wanted to share:

"I am 63 years old and I developed Bronchitis in April 2018. After 10 days I went back to a walk-in clinic and they said my lungs were clear, but I was in AFIB. They sent me to the ER where I was admitted for testing. Two days later I was diagnosed with AFIB and Stage 3 CHF with an EF of 20%. They did a second Echocardiogram and it came out with an EF% of 22. It took another 5 days to regulate my heart rate and blood pressure. With all the meds listed above. The Meds eventually drove my BP down to where I would get dizzy when I stood up and would occasionally pass out. I was having a hard time getting information from my Drs. I had been switched to 3 different Cardiologists in 6 weeks and all I could get appointments for were their NPs. My wife and I decided to schedule appointments at the Cleveland Clinic (a 4-hour drive away) the quickest we could get in was 6 weeks out. After my 3rd and 4th episodes of passing out we went over 2 days early and I was admitted through their ER on Sunday After meeting with 2 cardiologists on Tuesday and went through an Echocardiogram that showed my EF had improved to 48%. I have continued to diet and exercise as my youngest son says "like my life depends on it" I am now scheduled to go back to the Cleveland Clinic in 10 days for an Ablation Procedure that will take between 6 and 8 hours."

Thanks for sharing this story.

Lisa J.   Mio, MI   (#54)

Lisa has been part of our CHF world for 3 years.

The main symptoms she experiences are explained this way:

"Fatigue is huge. Often overwhelming. Frequent shortness of breath with little exertion, angina, extreme weight fluctuations, pressure on my chest, dizziness and recently memory loss."

CHF has impacted her quality of life described like this:

"It has slowed me down significantly. I'm only 42 but I feel much older. I have continued to try to work in my career as a nurse but I continue to go back into active CHF because of it. I make the best of the good days and try to rest on the bad days."

Lisa is being treated with medications:

"Diuretics-Demadex and Aldactone, potassium supplements to replace what the diuretics take away, beta blocker-Metoprolol succinate, antidepressants to deal with the emotional side of this disease."

She is experiencing Depression/ Anxiety described like this:

"Yes. I have always struggled with depression but the progression of the disease has only made it worse. I tend to have more anxiety at times when I'm not doing well physically. It affects my motivation and causes me to be

very introverted. I don't want to be social because no one understands my "invisible" disease."

She says the worst thing about CHF is:

"There is no cure."

This is the story she wanted to share:

"I started this journey in my twenties when I was experiencing a lot of heart palpitations and shortness of breath with activity. I was finally diagnosed with Hypertrophic cardiomyopathy (HCOM) with obstruction in 2007. No one really knew enough about it to educate me on how I should be monitored. Ended up in the hospital for 10 days because of that. So, I carried on for the next several years being monitored by a wonderful cardiologist at University of Michigan hospital. I had open heart surgery in 2012 to help alleviate the symptoms of HCOM but it was not a cure. I was feeling better for a couple of years but it went downhill again, this time leading to CHF. It has been a roller coaster ride for the past few years. I will keep fighting because I want to live a longer life and be a part of my children's lives."

Thanks for sharing this story.

Ellen   Fremont, CA   (#55)

Ellen is one of the more experienced members who has been part of our CHF world since 2004.

The main symptoms she experiences are explained this way:

"Fatigue, short of breath, water retention and heart rhythm issues"

CHF has impacted her quality of life described like this:

"The fatigue is debilitating. I can't exercise as needed and now I can't hold down a full-time job."

Ellen is being treated with medications:

"Entresto, Coreg, Lasix, potassium, Levothyroxine, Metformin, aspirin."

She is <u>not</u> experiencing Depression/ Anxiety.

She says the worst thing about CHF is:

"Impacts quality of life."

This is the story she wanted to share:

"My CHF was caused by chemotherapy drug Adriamycin. My ejection fraction seems to drop every time I get sick with a bronchitis or respiratory flu."

Thanks for sharing this story.

Mark W.   Wheeling, WV   (#56)

Mark has been part of our CHF world for 4 years.

The main symptoms he experiences are explained this way:

"Dizziness, shortness of breath, insomnia, weight gain (in spite of loss of appetite) and mild depression."

CHF has impacted his quality of life described like this:

"I find myself having to slow down. I still enjoy life, though!."

Mark is being treated with medications:

"Coreg, Lisinopril, Lipitor, CoQ10, magnesium, aspirin, a multi-vitamin, and Clonazepam (as needed) for restless leg syndrome."

He is experiencing Depression/ Anxiety described like this:

"Occasional (slight) depression/anxiety. Nothing to complain about."

He says the worst thing about CHF is:

"Shortness of breath and less energy than I'm used to having."

This is the story she wanted to share:

"My CHF may have been caused by a virus. More likely, due to excessive smoking (cigarettes) and drinking (vodka)."

Thanks for sharing this story.

Suzy H.   Spring, TX (#57)

Suzy has been part of our CHF world for 1 year.

The main symptoms she experiences are explained this way:

"Weight gain, Edema, memory loss, shortness of breath and depression."

CHF has impacted her quality of life described like this:

"CHF has totally turned my life upside down. I cannot work, shop, cook. clean, exercise or anything other than sit in my recliner and pray."

Suzy is being treated with medications:

"I take 24 different kinds of medication but that is because I have several other medical issue's other than CHF."

She is experiencing Depression/ Anxiety described like this:

"Yes! I feel like a burden to my family and society. I don't like to be around people anymore because I feel like everyone thinks I should be able to do more than I am able. I feel judged by all."

She says the worst thing about CHF is:

"The shortness of breath and the way it takes your life away."

She <u>did not</u> choose to share a life story.

Thanks for sharing this information.

Name Withheld   Asheville, NC   (#58)

This member has been part of our CHF world for 2 years.

The main symptoms they experience are explained this way:

"Fluid retention is my biggest challenge."

CHF has impacted their quality of life described like this:

"In some ways it's been good. I went on the low sodium diet and started going to the gym 5 to 6 days a week."

They are being treated with medications:

"Coreg, Spironolactone, Lisinopril, CoQ10, and fish oil daily. Lasix as needed."

They <u>do not</u> have issues with Depression/ Anxiety.

They say the worst thing about CHF is:

"Not knowing how the disease will changed."

This is the story they wanted to share:

"I started a blog, www.theunsaltytraveler.com to help me and others deal with life and travel with CHF."

Thanks for sharing this story.

Roxie A.   *Conklin, NY*   (#59)

Roxie has been part of our CHF world for just 1 year.

The main symptoms she experiences are explained this way:

"Fatigue, upset stomach, weight gain and now type 2 diabetes."

CHF has impacted her quality of life described like this:

"My home needs a good cleaning."

Roxie is being treated with medications:

"Fluid pills and Blood Pressure pills,"

She is <u>not</u> experiencing Depression/ Anxiety.

She says the worst thing about CHF is:

"It slowed me down.."

This is the story she wanted to share:

"Try to stay positive."

Amie K.   Florence, AL   (#60)

Amie has been part of our CHF world for the majority of her life.

The main symptoms she experiences are explained this way:

"Tiredness, swelling, dizzy all the time, I'm dyslexic it has made it worse. Shortness of breath. Episodes of major brain fog. And I get angry easier."

CHF has impacted her quality of life described like this:

"Turned my life upside down, I was a nonstop go-go kind of person, building my own business and CHF has been a brick wall..

Amie is being treated with medications:

"The usual heart failure cocktail, Coreg, Valsartan and Spironolactone."

She is experiencing Depression/ Anxiety described like this:

"Mainly Anxiety. I feel like my whole body could explode at any minute. I find simple things get on my nerves as where before they never bothered me."

She says the worst thing about CHF is:

"The getting worn out so easy and the fact that it has changed my life so much."

This is the story she wanted to share:

"I'm a 41 yr old active Female, three beautiful children 2 girls and 1 boy. Two are grown 26 and 19 one is still at home, he's 8. I watched my dad pass at a young age of 41 from CHF then my mother at 49. I knew I was doomed all my life, I have had heart trouble. Never got to play sports or do some of the fun things "normal" kids got to do. As I grew older, my problems didn't seem to grow with me, even though all my pregnancies, working and living. Moved to Alabama at 29 my husband's family are all from the area. And my youngest was born here with a little high blood pressure. Separated from my husband, and this is where my life really starts to go crazy. My estranged husband went to jail. He was caught robbing a bank. Well living in a small city the news of that spread like wildfire. I had separated from him a year earlier and the stress of that I had my first heart attack at 37. Son, you could only imagine my stress level now. Every and any kind of investigation agency was in my face, I don't know why but it almost gave me a nervous breakdown at that time but I managed to pick up and go on with what shred of normal life I had left, that was 2014. Met my new husband that fall of 2014 and was happy, life was good, the fire of the turmoil had just about burned out. Fast forward 2015, I fell in our pool and broke my tailbone, they don't treat tailbone breaks. I don't remember it hurting as bad when I was a kid but it took me down. I got sick on top of it all was told I had nothing wrong with me I was just being lazy. So, after going through episodes of not being able to get out of bed fighting with my doctors there's something wrong with me and being treated like I was a hypochondriac I got sick again in September 2017, this time I wasn't bouncing back something was bad wrong. My husband had also lost his job. We were about to lose our house so we decided to move into a house we had for rental in February 2018. I didn't have the strength to pack or move anything. Went to the ER and collapsed,

spent 5 days in the hospital was told I had COPD. Got home wasn't feeling any better at all, doctor told me I need to change my life style diet and exercise. Ok well I eat good my life style was as normal as could be. Exercise was out of the picture. I'm not being lazy but just walking to the mail box made me feel as if I was going to die. Maybe I'm crazy but definitely not lazy!! Got a new cardiologist and my life forever changed, he found it. I had a enlarged heart no blockage, no notable cause but it was there I had heart failure, the day I was diagnosed I came home to an empty house, my husband had left me, no job, no family, no money and a failing heart."

Thanks for sharing this story.

Jesse M.   *Las Vegas, NV*   (#61)

Jesse has been part of our CHF world for a year and a half.

The main symptoms she experiences are explained this way:

"Terrible stamina, mild shortness of breath and occasional lightheadedness."

CHF has impacted her quality of life described like this:

"I can't work. I can't sit for more than a couple hours at a time. I can't stand for a half an hour at a time. It is starting to make me feel down."

Jesse is being treated with medications:

"Carvedilol, Valsartan, Eliquis, Amiodarone, Furosemide, Lipitor, Gabapentin, Bupropion, Cimetidine, Vit D, Calcium, and Vit B."

She is experiencing Depression/ Anxiety described like this:

"Starting to. Everyone keeps talking about EF as if that tells the whole story of your condition. My EF is improving and my energy has slowly been improving, but my energy is still not good enough to work or do much except errands like grocery shopping and stopping at the drug store."

She says the worst thing about CHF is:

"I'm not living my life anymore. I had planned on working 9 more years. I don't think I'll ever be able to go back."

This is the story she wanted to share:

"I've been living over a year now without an income. Fortunately, I always enjoyed saving money. But now I'm spending down my money I expected to have for retirement and I haven't gotten approved for SSDI disability yet. I meant to work at least till full retirement age, so this has been a real shocker and depressing for me. I enjoyed my work and my coworkers. But I will cry if I get denied benefits and they say I can work again. I can't. I get sick feeling just trying to do 3 or 4 hours in a day of light upright activity. I have not done an 8-hour day since this happened to me. How could I possibly do 8 hours 5 days a week? If I get approved for SSDI, then I can care more about my health than about the state of limbo that I am in."

Thanks for sharing this story.

Leslie   *Clarksville, IN*   (#64)

Leslie has been involved in our CHF world since birth.

The main symptoms she experiences are explained this way:

"Edema, fatigue, weight gain and memory loss."

CHF has impacted her quality of life described like this:

"Very poor , can't do normal life activities like: hiking and taking long walks."

Leslie is being treated with medications:

"Blood pressure, blood thinner, cholesterol, potassium, depression, anxiety and diuretics."

She is experiencing Depression/ Anxiety described like this:

"Yes, especially anxiety I'm scared when I go the hospital I won't come home."

She says the worst thing about CHF is:

"Shortness of breath."

This is the story she wanted to share via e-mail:

"I was born on September 13,1981. I had multiple ASD's (atrial septal defect) and VSD's (ventricular septal defect). I had my first open heart surgery when I was just three months old, to repair some of the holes in my heart. At six months, I had another open heart to repair the rest. I had a g-tube also, because I couldn't swallow. My lungs also collapsed so they had to put tubes in my lungs to "inflate" them back up. I spent my first 9 months of my life in the NICU, here in Louisville, Ky. The doctors told my family with my heart and lungs the way they were when I was born I would not live past five years old. All throughout my child hood I was in and out of the hospital for my heart! Fast forward. To November 2002. I had my first child, I was put in the high-risk category due to my heart condition, with luck ever thing went smooth with having my son, even though I did have a C-section and was monitored very closely. After I had him I felt fine and was doing normal daily activities that I could do back then. In 2003, I got pregnant with my daughter had her in April of 2004, she was premature, because I got so big with her she put a lot of pressure on my heart and reopened one of my VSD's they had repaired when I was a baby. So right after I gave birth we spent a month and a half in the hospital due to my not wanting her to leave me while I had my heart surgery. On January 25,2012, I was driving I started feeling funny, drove right past a hospital, but kept going didn't even stop. I had told my son to hop in the front to pull the car over while I was driving. Well by the grace of God, we made it home safely, told both my kids I was going to just sleep it off I would be fine. My son freaked out and called my best friend to come get me and take me to the ER. Good thing she did, because that's the day I was having my first heart attack. I was rushed to Catheterization lab (family not with me yet, just my kids). They put four stints into my heart. I was ok after that. March of the same year I had another heart attack, but this time I was already in the hospital so back to Cath lab I went and got two more stents. I should also say through all of these events I was still being seen by my pediatric cardiologist. The summer of 2012, I got a phone call from the peds cardiologist and he referred me to the heart transplant center to be evaluated. I was a ball of nerves. When I started seeing them August of

2012, I will never forget the doc sent me straight to the hospital, because my color was green and it freaked him out. Yes, I was in there for the longest time until they got me stable. In October 2012, I received my St. JUDE ICD. At the time of the ICD my Ejection Fraction was 10% and now with the ICD it is just a little at 25%. I have not had a heart transplant. Fast forward to now. I am stable for the most part. I forgot to mention how cold I get. It was 75 degrees in the house and I had a cardigan over my top and was still cold. My heart often doesn't pump strongly enough to keep me warm. I try to push myself, but my kids get on me. I was truly blessed to have my son around when I did, because of him freaking out that day back in 2012 I am still here. I call him my angel. "

Thanks for sharing this story.

Jack K.   *Hutchinson, KS (#65)*

Jack is new to our CHF world and has been in the CHF world since diagnosed December 2017.

The main symptom he experiences are explained as:

"Fatigue."

CHF has impacted his quality of life described like this:

"You realize what is important and what's not."

Jack is being treated with medications:

"Lisinopril, carvedilol, Lasix and potassium."

He is experiencing Depression/ Anxiety described like this:

"Sometimes, have to remind myself, I'm not dead yet."

He says the worst thing about CHF is:

"Fatigue."

This is the story he wanted to share:

"Every day is a new battle to be won."

Thanks for sharing this story.

Chris T.   Sullivan, MO   (#66)

Chris has been a Caregiver in our CHF world and has been doing it for 10 years. (Caregiver's responses reflect the patient they are associated with.)

The main symptoms they experience are explained as:

"Drastic weight gain, ridiculous amount of Edema, tired, short of breath, can't walk more than 20 feet without resting, stasis ulcers, hydrocele's (multiple times), fluid buildup around the heart and lungs, pneumonia and lymphEdema."

CHF has impacted their quality of life described like this:

"Sex life is non-existent. Former actives are no longer possible (playing sports with my kids, practicing, running, or even hiking). Super high bills as I am still working and not on disability yet. Medical terminology! I hate it...Acronyms! hate them too!"

They are being treated with medications:

"Metoprolol, Lisinopril, Lasix, Hydralazine, and 8 more...total of 12 several times a day."

They are experiencing Depression/ Anxiety described like this:

"Absolutely."

They say the worst thing about CHF is:

"Cannot even walk through Walmart without losing my breath and having to sit down! Not being able to play with my kids is the biggest!"

This is the story they wanted to share:

"Never smoked a day in my life. No drugs. no alcohol. All hereditary. My father past 4 years ago after having a heart attack (also CHF patient), then had 2 strokes within 2 weeks of having stints placed. He was only 61. I never really looked into what it meant to have CHF. I figured if it was that bad, one of my many Drs would explain it to me and tell me what I needed to do. It was not until my 2nd heart attack that my cardiologist said I might want to start slowing down and taking it easy. That was 8 years later. I was only 42. I dropped in full cardiac arrest in front of my 10-year-old daughter. So traumatic for her and for my wife. About 3 months ago, I got a "sore" on my leg. Started out as a scratch from the dishwasher door. Within weeks was a HUGE open abscess that I was to learn later was a Stasis ulcer. My feet and legs swell to more than double their size. Dark purple in color and ALWAYS extremely painful. Drs tell me to be as active as I can, then follow it with 'keep your feet elevated as much as possible"! I sure wish they would make up their mind. Having a loving supportive spouse makes all the difference in the world."

Thanks for sharing this story.

Name Withheld Brighton, TN (#67)

This member has been in the CHF world for 6 years, but has had symptoms before that.

The main symptoms they experience are explained as:

"Occasional weight gain and Edema. Some short-term memory loss, shortness of breath with exertion. Tired, body often feels weak (this is recent)."

CHF has impacted their quality of life described like this:

"While I have been able to do a lot, I have had to retire at 59. I miss working with the patients and their families."

They are being treated with medications:

"Lasix, Coreg, Bidil, Spironolactone, Levothyroxine, Losartan, Plavix, aspirin , Pepcid and 3 other meds for my stomach, vitamins(all prescribed by doctors), Insulin via Insulin pump."

They are not experiencing Depression/ Anxiety.

They say the worst thing about CHF is:

"How it affects the entire body, especially the kidneys."

This is the story he wanted to share:

"I had a history of shortness of breath and tiredness for several years. I was found to have sleep apnea and started using a CPAP which helped the tiredness. Aug 12, 2012, I had Angina. Initially pain left upper arm, then mid chest, finally my jaw. By the time the paramedics arrived, I had no pain, BP was 170s/ low 100s. Literally after 2 minutes in the ambulance I had a cardiac arrest. On arrival at hospital I was taken straight to the Catheterization lab where they saw my LAD (Left Anterior Descending) collapse and I was shocked for the 3rd time. I had emergency bypass surgery. Due to this episode, I had an EF of 30%. Over time it improved to 40 to 45%. I have been hospitalized twice since Aug 2012 with CHF. The first time was due to Anemia, the second time I had 14 pounds of fluid removed with IV Lasix, my EF dropped to 30% and I was given an AICD. A year ago, my EF was stable at 40 to 45% again. I have remained as active as possible with rehab, travel etc. I try not to let CHF hold me back."

Thanks for sharing this story.

Robert B.   Annan, Dumfries and Galloway, UK (#68)

Robert has been in our CHF world for 6 years.

The main symptoms he experiences are explained as:

"Weight gain, dizziness, tired most of the time and depression."

CHF has impacted his quality of life described like this:

"Unable to work, not able to lead the life I had."

Robert is being treated with medications:

"Inspire, Amiodarone, Bisoprolol, aspirin, Allopurinol and Entresto."

He is experiencing Depression/ Anxiety described like this:

"Feel low, not wanting to talk to anyone or go out."

He says the worst thing about CHF is:

"The unknown."

This is the story he wanted to share:

"Born 1964 with TOF (Tetralogy of Fallot) had correction 1968. Led an active lifestyle until 2011 when heart decided it had enough. Had a valve fitted 3 months later got another valve due to a growth on the last one had an ICD fitted 2014, had an Ablation which help to stop ICD shocking me. In 2016 had device changed to CRT-D and started on Entresto now it helps not as many abnormal rhythms. Sorry not technical I leave that to doctors."

Thanks for sharing this story.

Name Withheld Kalamazoo, MI   (#69)

This member is a Caregiver in our CHF world for less than 1 year (Caregivers have been asked to provide answers as the patient.)

The main symptoms they experience are explained as:

"Weight gain, Edema, breathlessness and fatigue."

CHF has impacted their quality of life described like this:

"Harder to watch our grandchildren, hard to walk and changed our diet and food intake greatly. We now have large bills from the hospitalization."

They are being treated with medications:

"Meds for HTP (Heart Transplant Patients), arrhythmia, blood thinner, Lipitor, Metformin and Lasix"

They are experiencing Depression/ Anxiety described like this:

"He suffers from some anxiety. Can be negative or lash out at family members verbally, not the grandkids though very loving with them mostly. Feels home bound somewhat isolated. Had to retire earlier than hoped for."

They say the worst thing about CHF is:

"Getting used to diet and fluid restrictions. Worries about money costs to it."

This is the story he wanted to share:

"Was diagnosed with blockages and arrythmia at age 53. Stents were done but heart beat never returned to normal after many years. Working a busy stressful job. Took meds saw cardiologist but never did rehab center for exercise. 10 years later (or less but not caught in beginning) had breathlessness, fatigue, Edema and weight gain. Not caught by cardiologist for over a year! Ended up in ER and finally diagnosed with CHF. Lost almost 40 pounds in Hospital over next 5 days on IV Lasix. Now 1 month later still losing weight on 2000 kcal diet, 2000 mg Na and 2000ml fluid and doing well but it is hard to maintain when traveling, trying to eat out or get take in food, or with multigenerational family members. He's doing it and doing very well but it can be tough and he's a very good cook. Experimenting with herbs and spices but that's not for everyone. Son in law doesn't like the food here anymore! We do though. Stamina for exercise or activity still very low one month later. He still has to get sleep study done and they want him to see a vascular specialist for his legs but he worries about co pays and money and bills. He's in the CHF clinic now at Bronson hospital. Needs a new cardiologist which they are aware of. How did this get missed by his last one for so long until he's in the ER?! He's trying to still go camping and some fun things with family and we did it but cannot tolerate heat well at all. He is not part of this FB group but I am (spouse) for info ideas and to hear people's stories. Some are much worse than ours that's for sure."

Thanks for sharing this story.

Name Withheld   Sanford, NC   (#70)

This member is a Caregiver in our CHF world for about 1 year (Caregivers have been asked to provide answers as the patient.)

The main symptoms they experience are explained as:

"Shortness of Breath, Edema and memory loss."

CHF has impacted their quality of life described like this:

"Can't pursue my hobbies—rebuilding motorcycles, long distance riding, other motorcycle related activities."

They are being treated with medications:

"7 for BP and heart, statin, insulin, Uloric and Prednisone"

They are experiencing Depression/ Anxiety described like this:

"Both. Drains my energy, drives my wife crazy."

They say the worst thing about CHF is:

"Loss of energy."

This is the story they wanted to share:

"Stage 4 kidney failure rules out many of the usual interventions. Salt was my favorite food."

Thanks for sharing this story.

Ciara B.   Triangle, VA   (#72)

Ciara has been in our CHF world for 3 years.

The main symptoms she experiences are explained as:

"Feet swelling, tired walking on a humid day, memory loss and weight gain."

CHF has impacted her quality of life described like this:

"Have to be more careful on humid days, take my shoes off at the end of the day, water pills hard on my weak bladder, watch out for signs that the condition is worsening, My short term memory is weaker"

Ciara is being treated with medications:

"Take 4 classic heart meds, 2 are water pills, Also take thyroid medicine, antidepressants and bladder medicine."

She is experiencing Depression/ Anxiety described like this:

"Had depression & anxiety prior to CHF. Started taking antidepressants after cancer. Have a rare condition called Cowden's. I just turned 44. CHF at first felt like a nail in my coffin, but now it is a another step in my journey .."

She says the worst thing about CHF is:

"Feeling like it can get worse easily and it is always part of my life."

This is the story she wanted to share:

"My mother had Cancer, Cowden's, CHF, Diabetes and more, but managed to still slay life's dragons till about 5 years ago when heaven decided she should rest. She set a great example to keep fighting. My dad set a great example that you support those who you love who are fighting. My dad was in the Military so we lucky to travel to Germany, England and Okinawa. We settled in Virginia near relatives. I am and was a Shy person so it is almost always a challenge to stand up for myself. I had my thyroid removed in 1997. I got cancer in 2000. I got a nice position helping with paperwork at social services in 2001. I am still at social services. I am lucky they helped with my ailments but struggle with the job. I am a shy single lady. Found out about my rare condition Cowden's about 2012. About 3 years ago, I thought I had a bad cold. Turned out to be much worse. Turned out to be heart failure. A brief coma, lots of healing and I am lucky to be semi-healthy, knock on wood. Struggle with water pills but do ok. Looking forward to keeping up the fight."

Thanks for sharing this story.

Sandy P.   *Oklahoma City, OK*   *(#73)*

Sandy has been in our CHF world for 1 year.

The main symptoms she experiences are explained as:

"Constant fighting to maintain a reasonable weight. Edema, always dizzy, pain on my left side."

CHF has impacted her quality of life described like this:

"I am out of breath and can not complete most chores with out rest. I sleep about 18 hours a day. I have little desire to even leave my house. I have one good day and 10 bad ones. I think my family is tired of my lifestyle."

Sandy is being treated with medications:

"Diuretic, Beta Blocker, Xanax, ACE Inhibitor and Zoloft."

She is experiencing Depression/ Anxiety described like this:

"I am suffering from both. That is why I am on Zoloft and Xanax. I can not physically do the things I need to do. It seems to be getting worse rapidly."

She says the worst thing about CHF is:

"The depression and the knowledge that it is progressive."

This is the story she wanted to share:

"I thought I had a cold, 3 weeks later I was still coughing. I had a chest X-ray and they found plural effusion. On follow up Echo it was determined I was in stage 2 of Diastolic Heart Failure. Everything I do is an effort. My husband does not realize this is serious. He is very unhappy that I go to sleep on every drive or event we go to. My friends don't understand that I can't do things like I could last year or even last month."

Thanks for sharing this story.

Martin A.   Birmingham, West Midlands, England   (#74)

Martin has been in our CHF world for 2 years.

The main symptoms he experiences are explained as:

"Chest Pain and Fatigue."

CHF has impacted his quality of life described like this:

"Has changed my life. Totally change my diet and can't do as much as I use too."

Martin is being treated with medications:

"Amiodarone, Aspirin, Atorvastatin, Furosemide, Ramipril, Spironolactone and Bisoprolol. Every single day for rest of my life. I'm 34."

He is experiencing Depression/ Anxiety described like this:

"I did suffer depression/ anxiety when I first was told I had heart failure but as I stick to my routine everyday, showed me, I have got better and that if I stick to this routine of tablets and being my careful with sugar and salt, I will be okay. I do have bad days but they never last."

He says the worst thing about CHF is:

"The chest pains and the fatigue. Feeling always tired."

This is the story he wanted to share:

"It started as I thought I had bad indigestion and I could walk 5 feet without being out of breathe. Went to doctor and they said it was my heart and it's very serious. I rested at home with tablets but got worse so went in hospital where they told my ECG test read 210/140 while sitting perfectly still so I had echocardiogram which show my left side of my heart was 15% active. Spent 9 days in hospital which did save my life, I've had to change my life around but if I could tell anyone being told the news I had. "Yes it is very serious but things will get better, I promise."

Thanks for sharing this story.

Dianne G. (#75)   *Langley, British Columbia, Canada*

Dianne said she has been diagnosed with CHF for about 7 years, but may have had it for much longer.

The main symptoms she experiences are explained as:

"It's hard for me to separate CHF symptoms from the symptoms of other diseases that I have. What I know for sure is the swelling in my legs and abdomen, cough and fatigue are from CHF."

CHF has impacted her quality of life described like this:

"I have to say no so many times. I have to say no to my husband, to my children and to myself. I often can't join in family outings or activities. I can't go grocery shopping some days. Cooking can be an issue - often my husband has to take over so many household chores. Not being able to participate with my family because I'm tired is heartbreaking. I've spent many days/nights too tired to cry over my disappointment."

Dianne is being treated with medications:

"Again, it's hard for me to separate my other medical issues here. I take Furosemide for the fluid gain, that much I know is from the CHF.."

She talked about Depression/ Anxiety like this:

"No, although the issues are depressing I just have to have my pity party for an hour or so, then pick myself up, dust myself off and carry on.."

She says the worst thing about CHF is:

"That it takes all my energy and that takes me away from my family.."

This is the story she wanted to share:

"I don't know when I developed heart failure, all I know is that when the Dr told me that's what I had that I remembered my Dad and how it affected him. What I knew is that heart failure changes your life and is life threatening.

I instantly had to make changes. I had to limit my fluid to 6 cups (1 1/2 litres) a day - that includes fruit, jello, soup, anything that has a liquid in it. My salt intake was lowered to 1500 mg a day. That involves everything else, bread, butter, mayo, chicken - everything. My social life became difficult, eating out was a nightmare of preparing ahead of time, checking on line for information regarding the food I was hoping to eat and finding out in most cases that my options were severely limited.

I've always been a bit of a defiant person - don't tell me what to do, I'll figure it out myself. Sometimes that's just not a good thing. Choosing to ignore my Dr's orders brought me to a rude awakening. I was taken to the ER because I was having problems breathing. I remember waking up in bed and sitting up gasping for oxygen, it felt like I was drowning. The first and second time that I was admitted for heart failure blend into each other. That's another problem I have, because my heart isn't pumping at full capacity oxygen doesn't fully reach my brain. There's enough to function, but I developed what's called brain fog and have a problem sorting things out properly. This can be awful, once it was so bad that I behaved selfishly and damaged an important relationship. (I remembered conversations far differently than others.)

Anyway, I do remember my ankles and feet swelling so badly that I had to wear slippers out in public for weeks. I couldn't walk more than a couple of minutes without stopping and gasping for air. Cleaning my house was too much for me so my husband had to take over and I had no energy at all for cooking (one of my passions). Basically I sat at my computer playing games on it and watching tv. Day and night. That was my life.

The third time that things became horrible I was on my dream vacation in Europe. We had decided to take a cruise ship rather than drive through the countries because I could be promised that my meals would be low sodium in the dining room of the ship. Well, I thought I was taking care of myself with just a few cheats but I continued to swell up and things became more and more difficult for me and once again I was unable to lie down in bed and breathe at the same time. I had to sit on the edge of the bed gasping for air and tell my husband that he had to take me to the medical office of the ship in the middle of the night because I couldn't breathe.

They didn't do much for me because their office is limited so the next morning we docked in Malta and I was taken off by stretcher into a waiting ambulance. I spent two weeks in Malta in a hospital room while my husband had to navigate the hotels and restaurants by himself. He rented a hotel room and spent most of the time at the hospital with me, so neither of us saw this beautiful Island. As a matter of fact, I spent my 60th birthday in a room with 5 other women from Malta, not with my family as I had planned.

Two weeks later I was taken by medivac back to a hospital near my home where I spent another week. The entire time I had problems breathing and was so tired - just weary. Eating required effort. I remember someone from one of the heart clinics coming in to talk to me and explaining how heart failure was affecting my heart. I have Diastolic Heart Failure, which means my heart is stiff, it doesn't pump the blood through and the worse my heart failure gets, the stiffer my heart will become until it won't be able to work any longer. That's scary. That is what made me decide to sit up and take notice. Ridiculous isn't it that I would take this so lightly for so long. I guess I'm the dimmer bulb in the chandelier. I'm sure that I had been told this information before, my Dr's *are very good at keeping me informed but for whatever reason, brain fog possibly, it didn't all sink in until then.*

I also have Atrial Fibrilation (AFIB) and have had to be cardioverted several times. AFIB is when my heart is beating erratically. I don't mind feeling the rapid heartbeat, it's the consequences of it that are so hard to deal with. The not being able to breathe is the worst for me. Once while in AFIB, I had a shower, trying to get dressed took me an entire hour because I had to lie down on the bed and rest and catch my breath after I put on each article of clothing. Cardioversion is another thing. The medical staff (sometimes ambulance drivers, sometimes nurses and sometimes technicians) attach a flat, flexible patch about 6 inches by 4 to the front and back left side of my chest, this is attached by wires to a machine. An IV has been started already and they deliver an anesthetic to knock me out then shock my heart back into regular rhythm. Sometimes it works on the first try, sometimes the second or third. Sometimes it doesn't work at all then a procedure called Ablation may be perfomed. I have had this, the Dr placed a catheter through my groin into my heart and burned spots that were causing the AFIB. I must say I have had more fun, but it was necessary and we all hoped this would work. It did for a few months, unfortunately my AFIB has come back, so now they want to give me a pacemaker. A little machine placed inside my chest with a wire to my heart. It's supposed to regulate the heart rate. I have to say that this scares me. A lot of things have happened and I have tried to have a positive attitude, because I am a firm believer in it making a difference. I think I'll have to work hard on that this time. Oh well, what's another challenge?

I manage day to day with heart failure. Some days are good, some not, things change constantly. Mostly I can't walk a full block, housework is done is 10 minute increments and I try to cook supper with my husband. There's the pain throughout my body, coughing, shortness of breath, AFIB, the constant blood work that I endure, the medical tests and procedures. My social life is almost nonexistent. Some friends understand when I don't talk to them for months at a time or I have to cancel at the last minute, some don't. What bothers me is that they think badly of me for the lack of attention they get. When it takes all my energy to take care of myself during the day and that's all I can do, well, that's all I can do.

Thankfully my children have supported me. They fill in the holes in my life with their love and caring. I'm much more fortunate than others and thank God every day for them.

I don't know how long I have to live with this disease, but none of us know how long we have to live anyway. I'm just going to try and get through it with a little grace, a lot of love and hopefully a smile."

Thanks for sharing this story.

Marcie B.   Shalimar, FL   (#76)

Marcie has been a Caregiver in our CHF world for 1 year. (Caregivers were asked to answer as the patient.)

The main symptoms they experience are explained:

"Weight gain and memory loss"

CHF has impacted their quality of life and described like this:

"At first she couldn't do anything, I mean anything!!!!!! Now she can."

They are being treated with medications:

"Metoprolol, Entresto, Eliquis, and Lasix. I think that's all may be wrong now because she's very intolerable of meds she took others weren't good."

Marcie's comment about experiencing Depression/ Anxiety:

"No !!! Actually I'm suffering"

Marcie said their worst thing about CHF is:

"I wouldn't know !! But I would have to say change in life style because that is what's hardest on me."

This is the story they wanted to share:

"Her story started 3 years ago she has been fighting Lyme! But hey I noticed something and I kept saying please go see a doctor or go through ER she would go through stages like she would be so pale and on the verge of passing out this has happened on several occasions enough to scare the hell out of me!! My wife is very very hard headed anyway I would go into more detail but it's late."

Thanks for sharing this story.

Janet L.   Brooklyn, NY   (#77)

Janet has been in our CHF world for 1 year.

The main symptoms she experiences are explained as:

"Edema, some memory loss and dizziness."

CHF has impacted her quality of life described like this:

"I am unable to complete as many items in a day as I would have in the past. I have to stop and take deep breaths quite often."

Janet is being treated with medications:

"Metoprolol."

She is experiencing Depression/ Anxiety described like this:

"Yes, I suffer from anxiety which becomes more severe, as I live alone.."

She says the worst thing about CHF is:

"Changes life expectancy."

This is the story she wanted to share:

"I am a 42 year old single woman recently diagnosed with Heart Failure. I suffered from sever swelling in my feet, legs and stomach which led me to be hospitalized. Everyday since my diagnosis I live in fear of my life. I feel lost, confused and hurt. I have been able to find this group and in the short time that I have been a member, I have learned so much and have less anxiety regarding my diagnosis and for that I am grateful.."

Thanks for sharing this story.

Daniel D.   Ravenswood, WV   (#78)

Daniel has been in our CHF world for 6 years.

The main symptoms he experiences are explained as:

"Dizziness, memory, out of breath bending over and fatigue."

CHF has impacted his quality of life described like this:

"Eating right cut out, salt pacing myself. working out sometimes, I feel like a broken superman"

Daniel is being treated with medications:

"Entrestro, Brilinta, potassium, Atorvastati, Metroprolol, Pantoprazole, nitro glycerin, furosemide and asprin."

He is not experiencing Depression/ Anxiety.

He says the worst thing about CHF is:

"Knowing you can't do what you use to do and always wondering when is the next time."

This is the story he wanted to share:

"In 2013 had 99% blockage widow maker, no damage 1 stent. In 2017 was coming home from work felt a massive one coming on. I could of turned around went hospital, did not think I would make it so I drove home to tell family I loved them and my wife called 911 ambulance. Met us at park and ride 17 mins later I am in the trama unit getting prepared for surgery 2 1/2 hours later I'm in my hospital room, I found out had a massive blood clot blocked my previous stent, 100% blockage and lost 1/3 of my heart. My EF was 15%. I wore a lifevest for 3 months brought it up to 45 - 50%.."

Thanks for sharing this story.

Name Withheld   Enfield, United Kingdom (#79)

This member has been in our CHF world just since April 2018.

The main symptoms they experience are explained as:

"I was diagnosed with CHF and Edema at the end of April 2018. I've had my good days and bad days. This weekend 02/09 was a complete disaster. I have been terrified, crying, anxious, nervous and my fingernails were very long and I have broken them and continue to pick them and the skin which I have occasionally picked and tore my finger skin off.."

CHF has impacted their quality of life described like this:

"I have not adjusted to having CHF. I can't get my head round it that I have this disease and Edema."

The member is being treated with medications:

"I have innumerable meds for many ailments including three types of diuretics pills to help with Edema.."

They are experiencing Depression/ Anxiety described like this:

"Yes, I am suffering depression and anxiety, tension, and, stress because I can NOT get my head round that I have CHF and Edema, particularly the former.."

They say the worst thing about CHF is:

_____

"I'm terrified that I'm going to have a coronary or just drop."

_____

This is the story they wanted to share:

_____

"I was only diagnosed four (4) months ago and so far, there hasn't been a lot of journey."

_____

Thanks for sharing this story.

Keith S.   *Kinghorn, Fife, Scotland*   *(#80)*

Keith has been in our CHF world for 2 years.

The main symptoms he experiences are explained as:

"Fatigue, memory loss, weight gain and shortness of breath."

CHF has impacted his quality of life described like this:

"I try not to let it get the better of me but I can't do all that I want to do or used to do. it gets depressing a lot of the time"

Keith is being treated with medications:

"Statins, aspirin, Losartan, Bisoprolol, Clopidogrel, Ranitidine, Lansoprazole."

He is experiencing Depression/ Anxiety described like this:

"Definitely I find I am getting less and less interested in life in general."

He says the worst thing about CHF is:

"The worst thing for me is not socialising as often as I used to I miss the old me the one who was always laughing and joking."

This is the story he wanted to share:

"I started off being told that I had COPD and was given inhalers that did very little for me. Then I was sent for tests which came back as needing more testing so I was sent to the main hospital where they found I had several blockages. The day I was booked in to have stents fitted, I was told that because the blockages were so severe I had to have CABG x 3, waited for a week to have this done everything seemed to go great, but an hour after the operation I had a massive heart attack thank god for the great nurse I had who managed to get my heart going again before they took me back through to operate again as the grafts had collapsed and had to be done again. I don't know if I was dreaming but I swear I could see the surgeon taking the artery out of my leg and everyone rushing around I had bad dreams about that for months. Today I'm just in a sort of low point as I feel useless. I can't walk far, I can't lift the things I used to and can't work. It makes it seem so pointless at times if it weren't for my family I honestly think I would have given up already."

Thanks for sharing this story.

Joe N.　　　Orland Park, IL　　(#81)

Joe has been in our CHF world for 5 years.

The main symptoms he experiences are explained as:

"Tiredness and slight dizziness at times."

CHF has impacted his quality of life described like this:

"I am 68yrs old and it has not impacted my life too much. I still go to the office almost every day and go out with friends a couple nights a week."

Joe is being treated with medications:

"Entresto, Amiodorone, Lipitor, Plavix, Aspirin, Ambien, Lasix and Coreg."

He is experiencing Depression/ Anxiety described like this:

"I have suffered anxiety since I was a teenager so it has nothing to do with CHF. Not depressed at all."

He says the worst thing about CHF is:

"Fatigued, Tiredness. Not eating what I want. Not being able to plan things because I do not know how I am going to feel that day."

This is the story he wanted to share:

"I had a stroke in 2013 and was diagnosed then, EF was 40% back then and dropped to 15% in the 5 years. Dr tells me that my heart muscle is very damaged and there is a chance it will not improve. Before I had a stroke I did have symptoms that I avoided. Short-of-breath, nosebleeds, insomnia, weight gain .. I did wear the vest for 60 days and I really did not like it so I sent it back. When my EF dropped to 25% I got a CRT and so glad I did because it did help me with my energy and fatigue. I do ok with CHF because I have had it long enough to know my limits. It takes time to settle in and learn your limits."

Thanks for sharing this story.

Sara B.   *Mt. Laurel, NJ*   (#82)

Sara has been in our CHF world for 2 years.

The main symptoms she experiences are explained as:

"Fatigue, Edema and achy."

CHF has impacted her quality of life described like this:

"I have lost strength and I can't do what I used to do with out stopping and catching my breathe. I take a lot of meds so I spend time tracking that."

Sara is being treated with medications:

"Norpace, Metoprolol, Coumadin, and a water pill are what I take for my heart. I take other meds that aren't cardiac related.."

She is experiencing Depression/ Anxiety described like this:

"Yes I take an antidepressant and if I think about it too much I burst into tears.."

She says the worst thing about CHF is:

"Being tired all the time and the meds!"

This is the story she wanted to share:

"Two years ago I ended up in the hospital with Afib and tachycardia. I ended up needing a pacemaker/defib. My doctor didn't want me to be pacemaker dependent, but it was unavoidable. I went back to the hospital with pneumonia and ended up in rehab to regain strength. While in rehab I started having trouble breathing and my legs swelled. That was when I was diagnosed with CHF. It really scared me because I thought I was going to die. I am very lucky to have my mom who is a retired nurse who helps me. I work full time but sometimes it is a struggle."

Thanks for sharing this story.

Isabelle D. Kitchener, Ont., Canada   *(#83)*

Isabelle has been in our CHF world since April of 2018.

The main symptoms she experiences are explained as:

"The biggest symptom is exhaustion I can't do anything here at home I couldn't be up for about five or 10 minutes and then I have to lay down or sit down at least."

CHF has impacted her quality of life described like this:

"I am trying not to let it affect my life I have other problems health problems as well so with the combination of all five things going on I have tried not to let the CHF get to me. I had an ICD implanted on July 30 and that makes me feel safer. I wasn't really worried because I don't believe in worrying but that certainly let me know that my life could possibly be extended. I couldn't do much before I was diagnosed and I don't do much now because my kids won't let me, I cook for myself and that's it"

Isabelle is being treated with medications:

"I take heart medication, blood thinners, antidepressant medication, medication for my fibromyalgia and medication for my rheumatoid arthritis and my osteoporosis and I think that's it."

She is not experiencing Depression/ Anxiety and said this:

"No I am not suffering from depression or anxiety because of CHF. I believe that it's in gods hands not mine so there's no point in me worrying about something that I can't change or I have no say over."

She says the worst thing about CHF is:

"I think the worst for me is not being able to take care of my own apartment as far as cleaning and things like that."

This is the story she wanted to share:

"My problem started about I think it's eight years ago I had my first heart attack I did not know I was having a heart attack because the only symptoms I had were I felt like I was getting the flu, but my daughters insisted I go get checked in at that time. I was having a heart attack from then I had a lot of issues the medications. It took them a long time to get them straightened out and the Lasix cost me a lot of the issues. I had dizzy spells I fell down all the time my kids finally move me back to my hometown, before that I had a spell when I just felt I was getting the flu, but I didn't go to the doctor or anything. I just ignored it that was about two years after my first heart attack. I move forward now to 2018 I had an pneumonia and went and had it checked, took antibiotics felt better. Weeks later got pneumonia again and at this time I could not keep fluid or anything in my stomach. I was throwing up everything and then I started urinating without any warning it just came and then my bowels started to do the same thing. I then of course got pneumonia again I went to the clinic because my son-in-law insisted I go to the walkin clinic. I did that and I was diagnosed with pneumonia again I went home to my daughters my son-in-law wanted me to go to ER. I of course didn't want to go but they made me . I could not inhale one breath when I got to the emergency room they checked me in right away and the doctor said you're having a

heart attack and are in heart failure. He told my daughter that I had possibly 10 minutes to live when they brought me in and that possibly I wasn't going to come out of this heart attack, but thank God I did. I was in the hospital for about a week they got rid of all the fluid I was retaining. I had fluid in my lungs and fluid around my heart. I came home with their restrictions on salt and liquid so I keep track of that every day, everything that I consumed gets written in my little book and I feel fine other then I have this horrible dry cough and I think that's the end of my story thank you."

Thanks for sharing this story.

Patricia R.   Dentin, MD   (#84)

Patricia has been in our CHF world for 2 1/2 years.

The main symptoms she experiences are explained as:

"I also have COPD so my diagnosis was delayed by a month. My youngest daughter went into premature labor and we headed to the hospital. I was so very SOB, I needed a wheel chair. After the baby and daughter came home, I decided enough was enough. I took myself to local ER, now thinking it was COPD. I suggested that they do a CT scan. Maybe plural effusion. They ordered an echo and found out my ef was only nine. Hospital (Anne Arundel medical center) I needed to go to was on code black and they would be sending me to Easton Memorial Hospital. I told them I would drive myself there. My other daughter just happened to be working as a tech on heart and vascular floor. There was a bed opened and I was direct admitted where I remained for ten days and 30 pounds lighter. My next Echo showed EF was 16. On all kinds of meds and water pills. Last two Echos EF was 50/55. "

CHF has impacted her quality of life described like this:

"Never thought about dying until this. I babysit my four grandkids (ages 2 to 7). I don't want them to grow up without me. As of now I am in recovery, since there isn't a cure for CHF. I take one day at a time. Unfortunately I still don't know the difference between CHF and COPD. While in hospital they also determined I was a type one diabetic. I also have bilateral kidney stones. Good part is I have lost another 15 pounds. I started out weight 170 pounds and today I was 115 pounds and am 5'5"."

Patricia is being treated with medications:

"Digoxin, Metoprolol and low dose aspirin."

She is <u>not</u> experiencing Depression/ Anxiety and said:

No. I guess I'm lucky

She says the worst thing about CHF is:

"Not being able to do everything I used to enjoy. Didn't feel confident enough to get into the ocean alone. Walking without having to rest.."

This is the story she wanted to share:

"My then 4 year old granddaughter came to visit me. She thought I was going to die and didn't want to leave me. I promised her I would do everything the doctors told me so I would be at the birthday party. I was discharged the day before her party.."

Thanks for sharing this story.

Kara H.　　　*Apple Valley, CA*　　　*(#85)*

Kara has been in our CHF world for a little over 2 years.

The main symptoms she experiences are explained as:

"Tired, weak, memory loss, dizzy and mild chest pains."

CHF has impacted her quality of life described like this:

"I have had a decline in my overall health. After I found out I had CHF my kidneys failed and I am on dialysis. I can no longer drive, work or go out of the house on my own. Before we got the dizziness under control I fell a lot. I now have a bed rail, shower chair, and my husband had tall toilets installed so I could get off the toilet on my own. He got Alexa so if I need help and can't call out I can ask her to call his office down the hall. I can't cook or decorate the house for the holidays, I can not shop for gifts the way I used to. I have sleep issues. I either can not get to sleep or I sleep 9 hours."

Kara is being treated with medications:

"Torsemide, Dilt-XR, Atorvastatin, phosphorus binder, Trazadone, and we are going to start looking for a b.p med that works but will not drop my b/p after dialysis."

She is experiencing Depression/ Anxiety described like this:

"I get anxiety when I need to ask for help. I still want to be independent and it's hard to ask for help. I get clammy, sweaty, nervous, dizzy and nausea.."

She says the worst thing about CHF is:

"Loss of independence."

This is the story she wanted to share:

"I worked in a cardiology dept. In December of 2015. I purchased a pair of shoes for our Christmas party, a day or two later I tried them on with the outfit I wanted wear. The shoes did not fit they were to small. I thought I brought home the box. I returned the shoes and got a larger pair. The day of the Christmas party I got dressed. The shoes again did not fit. I had to wear a pair slippers to the party. I never had problems with alot of swelling, In January of 2016 I got an e-mail, our company was doing a weight loss challenge, every pound you lost they would donate one pound of food to a food bank. I thought great I could loose 15 pounds and donate to a great cause. I signed up and was on my way, I was on my way to gaining weight. I could not loose anything. I was gaining a few pounds a week. So I stopped the challenge, I felt like a complete failure, not only did I let my self down but I let a food bank down that hurt alot. My husband took me to the Hollywood Bowl to see David Gilmour. He gave me the tickets in January for my birthday. I was over the moon I was so happy. We made a day of it. We went up eary in the day to avoid traffic, we went to a museum then had a late lunch , then it was off to the bowl. It was heart breaking. I had a difficult time walking. It is mostly up hill. I was short of breathe, clammy, chest pains, anxiety over my condition afraid that at any moment I would need to be taken to the ER. I was not going to miss this concert it was a once in a life time chance to see David Gilmour.

We finely made it to our seats. My husband went and got us drinks. I got to have the full Gilmour experience. The best concert I have ever seen. My dreams came true that night. I was happy and complete, but I knew something was really wrong with me. When the concert was over we made our way out and to the buses. I fell 2 times before we got to the bus. My husband and total strangers had to help me up. I could feel the fluid in my legs, it was up to my thighs almost up to my hips, the skin was so tight I could hardly move my legs. When we got to the bus I fell into it and had to have help getting up. Then we did not have seats I was 47 years old and I felt like I was to young, or to vain to ask one of the young men if I could have there seat. They dopped us off in front of the parking structure on Hollywood blvd. I told my husband to go get our car. I did not think I would make it with out falling and he could not help me up by himself. This was on Friday, on Monday after work I went to our Urgent Care, I had to go to the next closes facility to have labs and a chest x-ray, I got there just in time to get in line for them to close, so I went across town had my labs and x-ray. The next morning I went back to Urgent Care to get my results I was admitted to the hospital. I had CHF. I was scared, confused and lost. I had more x-rays, labs, an Echo, a heart Cath, the works. I had no idea what to do next. My diet had to change, I had to reduce my fluid intake, go low sodium and reduce stress. Everything would be different. My heart Cath was on April fools day, I felt like it was a cruel cosmic joke. I knew at any moment someone was going to jump out and say just kidding. But that did not happen, So I took a deep breathe. I started a new life. I did not use salt. I have not added salt to my food or cooked with it since some time prior to my hospital stay. It was strange at first, but I felt I could control that so I did. I started reducing my fluid intake, something else I could control. I worked on my food, this was harder at first you need to read every label. I had been taking medication so I did not need to make any life changing alterations, so that was easy. I went to CHF classes, living with chronic condition classes and saw a nutritionist. In September, I was admitted because my hemoglobin was to low. Over the next 10 months I had 9 pints of blood, labs, X-rays, Echos, Thallium treadmill, fluid drained from my lungs 4 times, a bone marrow biopsy. I was in the hospital a minimum of once a month. Then I found out my kidneys had failed, I needed to start dialysis. I have had to stop working, driving, doing *everything for myself and depending on others for just about every thing. However, I am alive, I have a new day every day. I live in a time when we have medicine and dialysis and other things that make life a little easier then it would be just 30 -40 years ago, I plan on living the best life I can live one day at a time.*

Thanks for sharing this story.

Scott D.   *Wooster, OH*   (#86)

Scott has been in our CHF world for 6 years.

The main symptoms he experiences are explained as:

"Edema, dizziness, fatigue and chest pain.."

CHF has impacted his quality of life described like this:

"It's made work terrible, no sex life, always adjusting my medicine."

Scott is being treated with medications:

"Lasix, Lisinopril, Lipitor, Plavix, Coreg, Norvasc, Hydrodiuril and asprin."

He is experiencing Depression/ Anxiety described like this:

"Night time Anxiety, but under control now without medicine."

He says the worst thing about CHF is:

"Fatigue."

This is the story he wanted to share:

"*I was 37 and had a massive heart attack, 99% blocked, didn't get intervention for more than 3 hours. Should have clotted and died, but never knew I had a anti-clotting blood disorder. That basically saved my life till I made it to the Cath Lab. Total of 4 heart attacks and 3 stents later, I'm still alive! My heart is severely damaged so normal life is over. I still work a physical job, and take a bunch of medicine. Nitroglycerin all the time. I also have Cardiomyopathy, AFIB, Hemophilia C, fatigue, chest pain, no sex life, are just some of my problems living with CHF.*"

Thanks for sharing this story.

Gloria W.   Scott City, MO   (#87)

Gloria an experienced member has been in our CHF world for 15 years.

The main symptoms she experiences are explained as:

"Palpitations, shortness of breath, weight gain, insomnia, and heat intolerance with excessive sweating."

CHF has impacted her quality of life described like this:

"Has slowed me down a lot. Lack of endurance with physical exertion. I avoid situations that require a lot of walking."

Gloria is being treated with medications:

"Lasix, Spironolactone, Zocor, Sotalol, Sertraline, Pradaxa and Entresto.."

She is experiencing Depression/ Anxiety described like this:

"Anxiety from worrying if my heart is doing ok. I think it contributes to my insomnia."

She says the worst thing about CHF is:

"The inability to do things I used to do, and the uncertainty of what my medical situation will bring."

This is the story she wanted to share:

"Began in 1988, with heart attack and triple bypass surgery. Attended Cardiac Rehab, which helped me both physically and emotionally. Suffered severe depression after surgery. In Dec. of 1988, our 13 yr old son died as a result of punishment by his school teacher, which increased my stress immensely. I then returned to smoking for the next 20 years. Had 2nd heart attack in 2003 with angioplasty afterwards. Was then diagnosed with CHF in 2003. Treatment consisted of meds only at that point. Did relatively well until 2014, when I was admitted to hospital with what was determined to be CHF with irregular heartbeat, and received ICD implant. Again, did relatively well until May of 2018, when I went to ER with shortness of breath, and feeling like I was going to pass out. Echo showed EF of 20. At this point, my ICD was removed and replaced with CRT/D, and placed on Entresto, which appears to be helping. Am now feeling better, and seem to be improving yet.."

Thanks for sharing this story.

Maribel H.   Ocala, FL   (#88)

Maribel has been in our CHF world as a Caregiver for 8 months. (Caregivers were asked to answer as the patient.)

The main symptoms the patient experiences are explained as:

"Edema, pain, dizziness, nausea, weight gain for liquid retention, shortness of breath."

CHF has impacted their quality of life described like this:

"my quality of life now is bad, can't do things."

The patient is being treated with medications:

"Many for high blood pressure, Lasix, Plavix, potassium,."

They are experiencing Depression/ Anxiety described like this:

"Anxiety and can't be alone."

She says the worst thing about CHF is:

"All."

This is the story they wanted to share:

"The most important thing now is that the doctors don't care and they send you to a different specialist because no one wants to have the responsibility. For CHF they need to have a place with all the doctors there and were they check often for all the different issues that CHF bring, Cardiologist, Kidney, and few other doctors all there and discuss with the patient altogether the plan for the well-being of the patient and he can tell them what they feel. CHF is not for only one doctor. Is for a group of specialist."

Thanks for sharing this story.

David K.   Opelika, AL   (#89)

David is very experienced with CHF and has been in our CHF world for 28 years.

The main symptoms he experiences are explained as:

"Weight gain, Edema, memory loss, dizziness, pain and 2 strokes."

CHF has impacted his quality of life described like this:

"Ended my working career."

David is being treated with medications but says:

"Too many to list LOL."

He is experiencing Depression/ Anxiety described like this:

"Yes , Daily."

He says the worst thing about CHF is:

"Give out so easy..cant do the things I enjoy. Have to stay inside all summer cant take the heat.."

This is the story he wanted to share:

"Had my 1 stroke at 25 and was diagnosed with COPD which later turned out to be CHF. I do some better with my pacemaker."

Thanks for sharing this story.

Steve D.   *Franklin, TX*   *(#90)*

Steve is pretty new to our CHF world and has been here for 5 months.

The main symptoms he experiences are explained as:

"Shortness of breath and weight gain."

CHF has impacted his quality of life described like this:

"Can't do much of anything outside anymore"

Steve is being treated with medications:

"Furosemide and Spironolactone."

He is <u>not</u> experiencing Depression/ Anxiety.

He says the worst thing about CHF is:

"Waking up in the night with shortness of breath."

This is the story he wanted to share:

"We went camping out of town and attended a wedding. I got short of breath during the first night. It got better. We came home and I had shortness of breath off and on during the week. My wife convinced me to go to the ER. I had a heart attack with congestive heart failure. I underwent CABGx3. Did well until two months later. Went to the ER again. I was in CHF. They put in. Pacer/defibrillator. I've done pretty well since then. I have routine visits at the heart failure clinic."

Thanks for sharing this story.

Mandy   *Folkestone, Kent, UK (#91)*

Mandy has been in our CHF world for just 1 year.

The main symptoms she experiences are explained as:

"I suffer from fatigue, breathlessness and fluid retention. I'm often dizzy and can't walk far. Recently I've found that a stick helps."

CHF has impacted her quality of life described like this:

"CHF has made me almost housebound. I tend not have the confidence to go out alone and so only go out for appointments. I executed to improve gradually but it's just not happened."

Mandy is being treated with medications:

"Statins, beta blockers, blood thinners, diuretics, etc..."

She is experiencing Depression/ Anxiety described like this:

"I suffer from anxiety and depression which means that I don't get out or socialise much. Counselling had helped..."

She says the worst thing about CHF is:

"The exhaustion. I just run out of steam and that's that. I also hate that people don't get that I'm ill because I look OK."

This is the story she wanted to share:

"I've had Chronic Fatigue syndrome for about 20 years and expect not to feel well, but the Christmas before last I had a virus and became more and more exhausted and very depressed. In April I went to vote and although it was only a short walk I had to keep sitting down and developed chest pains. Next day I went to my gp because I had a persistent cough and she sent me straight into hospital. Turned out it was my heart and heart failure. I'm on loads of drugs and my EF has gone from 15-20% to 55%, which would be great if I felt well. I also have kidney failure and a lung problem.."

Thanks for sharing this story.

Nancy N.   Addison, IL   (#92)

Nancy has been in our CHF world for 3 years.

The main symptoms she experiences are explained as:

"Weight gain, dizziness and memory loss."

CHF has impacted her quality of life described like this:

"I have fatigue and I am not able to do as much as I use to. I feel I struggle both physically and mentally at different times."

Nancy is being treated with medications:

"Coreg, Lisinopril, Spirolactone, Simivistatin and baby aspirin"

She is experiencing Depression/ Anxiety described like this:

"Yes I believe I am at times. Especially when I attempt to do something and am not able to anymore."

She says the worst thing about CHF is:

"The fatigue and not being able to be my best at times."

This is the story she wanted to share:

"I was diagnosed with non-Hodgkins lymphoma in 1996. Had years of chemo and had a bone marrow transplant in 2003. Had a recurrence of NHL in 2005. Was suffering from chronic graft vs. host disease but was dealing with it. Then in 2013 I found I was having trouble breathing. I hosted Easter dinner and that night I had fluid in my legs and feet. My father passed from CHF, so I knew it's symptoms but was hoping for a different outcome. Went to see my primary care physician who sent me for an Echo. He called me that night and when I realized it was my doc calling me I knew I had it before I even saw the cardiologist the next day. I have non ischemic, idiopathic CHF. Also found out I have non-compaction.."

Thanks for sharing this story.

Malcolm W. Swindon, Wiltshire, England (#93)

Malcolm has been in our CHF world for 12 years.

The main symptoms he experiences are explained as:

"Fatigue, breathlessness now but had many others."

CHF has impacted his quality of life described like this:

"Ruined it, stopped it and improved it."

Malcolm is being treated with medications:

"Take about ten a day but serious meds : My favourite Entresto, Carvedilol, Warfarin and two water tabs."

He is not experiencing Depression/ Anxiety described like this:

"No I deal with it.."

He says the worst thing about CHF is:

"Restrictions and shortness."

This is the story he wanted to share:

"I am a veteran patient of 23 years. My story begins when I was a super fit fanatic of 28 years old . More to say"

Thanks for sharing this story.

Kim Z.   Mason, OH   (#94)

Kim has been in our CHF world for 1 year.

The main symptoms she experiences are explained as:

"Weight gain, shortness of breath, Edema, memory loss and dizziness."

CHF has impacted her quality of life described like this:

"A big change, watching diet, more resting, someone else doing the housework, tired."

Kim is being treated with medications:

"Spironolactone, Carvedilol, vitamin D , aspirin, Claritian, Cymbalta and multi vitamin."

She is experiencing Depression/ Anxiety described like this:

"Depression and Anxiety - sleep or lack of it, worry, fear of not waking up ."

She says the worst thing about CHF is:

"Not feeling like my former self."

This is the story she wanted to share:

"HA/Widowmaker 4/29/17 one stent, systolic and diastolic heart failure, V Tach, ICD implant 8/7/17."

Thanks for sharing this story.

Angela D.   *Topeka, KA*   *(#95)*

Angela has been in our CHF world for 2 years.

The main symptoms she experiences are explained as:

"Weight gain, Edema, loss of hair growth on legs, jaw pain, whistling when breathing at night and shortness of breath."

CHF has impacted her quality of life described like this:

"A huge impact. I have no idea how long I've had this. I was only recently diagnosed and my life has changed significantly. Some days my life seems normal and other days simple things like laundry almost feel like an impossible task."

Angela is being treated with medications:

"Entresro, Carvedilol, Lasix, Atorvostatin, iron, vit d and b12. As well as Humalog and Levamir."

She is experiencing Depression/ Anxiety described like this:

"I have always suffered from anxiety and depression. It has definitely gotten worse since my diagnosis. I find myself focusing on how this will impact my life, how long do I have left to live, will I leave my 4 year old without a mother?.."

She says the worst thing about CHF is:

"The constant doctors appointments and lab work. The hardest thing for me to adjust to is the low sodium diet and water restrictions. I really miss just drinking what I want when I want. Also the shortness of breath. That makes even grocery shopping a chore."

This is the story she wanted to share:

"I got to the point that I was unable to walk from the couch to the bathroom with our being short of breath. My legs felt like there was concrete in them and I couldn't sleep without sitting up. I felt so alone and terrified and I knew that this is what I had, but coming to terms with actually hearing it was so hard. I was admitted for a week and lost 40lbs of fluid. Now I am on a journey to live."

Thanks for sharing this story.

David B.   Wales, MA   (#96)

David has been in our CHF world for 18 years.

The main symptom he experiences are explained as:

No Symptoms provided

CHF has impacted his quality of life described like this:

"Disabled young at 39, limited income stinks"

David is being treated with medications:

"Many, Lasix, BP"

He is experiencing Depression/ Anxiety described like this:

"Worthiness unable to contribute as once did."

He says the worst thing about CHF is:

"Loss of income, present and future."

This is the story he wanted to share:

"Survived 2 heart attacks, stroke and arthmia."

Thanks for sharing this story.

Jill T.   Dunnellon, FL   (#97)

Jill has been in our CHF world for 2 years.

The main symptoms she experiences are explained as:

"Weight gain, memory loss, dizziness and exhaustion."

CHF has impacted her quality of life described like this:

"I was very active and outgoing. Now my life has slowed down considerly."

Jill is being treated with medications:

"Entresto, 81 mg aspirin, Lasix, Metoprolol ER, Atorvastatin and Lexapro."

She is experiencing Depression/ Anxiety described like this:

"Depression. I think because I'm unable to do the things I did before."

She says the worst thing about CHF is:

"Breathing and lack of energy."

This is the story she wanted to share:

"I have 7 grandchildren that I adore. Not being able to play with them is heartbreaking. I've found new things to do with them, but things will never be the same."

Thanks for sharing this story.

Toni L.   *Smyrna, TN*   *(#98)*

Toni has been in our CHF world for just 1 year.

The main symptoms she experiences are explained as:

"Edema, Shortness of Breath and Dizziness."

CHF has impacted her quality of life described like this:

"Drastic loss of Income (can only work part time now) and Activity. I previously loved to travel and attend concerts but can no longer park and walk long distances (airport terminal & music venues) or do many stairs"

Toni is being treated with medications:

"Lasix, Coreg, Spironolactone and Lisinopril."

She is experiencing Depression/ Anxiety described like this:

"Somewhat but have come to grips with the condition and I'm trying to figure out how to enjoy and make my remaining years productive ...and fulfilling.."

She says the worst thing about CHF is:

"Inability to walk long distances and play with my grandbabies."

This is the story she wanted to share:

"tired, Tired, TIRED."

Thanks for sharing this story.

Kathy A.   Long Beach, CA   (#99)

Kathy has been in our CHF world about a year.

The main symptoms she experiences are explained as:

"Shortness of breath and Edema."

CHF has impacted her quality of life described like this:

"Driving restrictions and Dietary restrictions"

Kathy is being treated with medications:

"Amiodarone, Mexiletine, Bisoporal, Lasix, potassium, Lipitor and low dose aspirin."

She is experiencing Depression/ Anxiety described like this:

"Knowing how close I was to dying. I received an ICD, but then a week of 'storm' where it went off 5 times in the week and I was hospitalized again. I re-play these moments in my mind. The original episode and then the shocks."

She says the worst thing about CHF is:

"The uncertainty."

This is the story she wanted to share:

"In December of 2017, I had increasing shortness of breath and swelling. I had gone to a convention in Las Vegas and I could barely walk. At the end of that month, I was driving home from work and my heart just went. It was out of rhythm. I had to pull over to catch my breath. My husband has AFIB, so I am familiar with that. I wondered if I should call 911, go to the fire station (which was just up the block) or continue home. After some quick errands, I went home. I had called my husband to tell him that I wasn't feeling well. When I got home, he immediately drove me to the hospital. In the ER, they kept giving me meds to try and control my heart, but ended up having to shock me. This is all kind of blurry to me. When I did speak with the cardiologist at the hospital, he told me that I had been in VTAC and I would probably be receiving an ICD. This was all new vocabulary to me. He couldn't believe that I had driven in this state. Knowing what I know now, I should have called 911. I was then moved to another hospital with a specialized cardiac unit. After other test, I was given the ICD. I was in the hospital for 12 days. Then in April of this year, I was in the grocery store with my daughter. I could feel my heart racing and feeling horrible. My daughter was looking at me and could tell something was wrong. She asked if she could help me. Then my ICD fired. Wow! I flew down the aisle, knocked back. I then realized that my ICD was doing what it was supposed to do. It had just saved my life. The next night at home it went off again. And then the next day, I was at my office and it went off again. I was like, that's it. I had someone drive me to the hospital. While in the hospital, it fired 2 more times. I stayed in the hospital for a week. I was started on drips of Amiodarone and Mexiletine. I am now taking these as daily meds. Since that time, all has been quiet. There has been talk that one day I may have to have Ablation or even a transplant. I feel like I have entered a whole new world of terms. I understand the *seriousness that is VTAC. I know how close I was to death. It helps me to write poetry:*

I stare down death
One errant beat away
aware of the thin line of separation
the weight of a broken heart
~~~~
Who declared us enemies
You and I
Always trusting you secure
steadfast
dependable
now I live in fear
that trust shattered
O heart

Thanks for sharing this story.

Michael W.   Cleburne, TX   (#100)

Michael is another experienced member who has been in our CHF world for 18 years.

The main symptoms he experiences are explained as:

"Coughing, dizziness and memory loss,."

CHF has impacted his quality of life described like this:

"I'm not able to do things like I once was, I can't even work an easy part time job, I have had relationship problems, I can barely walk up my ramp that was built for me, I can't really pick anything up, I'm dependent on certain friends"

Michael is being treated with medications:

"Spirnolactone, Coreg, Digoxin, Furosemide, Entresto and Prozac"

He is experiencing Depression/ Anxiety described like this:

"Yes I have major anxiety, my depression is under control, my main issues right now are with my blood pressure, and shortness of breath at times."

He says the worst thing about CHF is:

"That I can't have a regular job, and stuck on a fixed income."

This is the story she wanted to share:

"Back in 2001, I started getting sick was constantly going to the ER. I was being misdiagnosed every single time told them the symptoms we're the same they were just getting worse, I was even kicked out of the ER by the Dr who told me to stop what I was doing and to get out of his ER. I finally got a call from the ER telling me to come back cause they finally looked at my x-rays and said my heart was enlarged. So I went back and all of a sudden I was in a high grade fever, couldn't stay awake and was told that all of my organs we're starting to shut down on me, from what my parents told me. I was in 2 hospitals for 10 days. The first hospital told me they wanted to send me to a different hospital because they didn't feel comfortable keeping me there, so after they got me stabilized and my fever of 107 went away I was transferred to Stanford University where I met my Dr that I would have for about 15 year, Dr. Randall Vagelos. With everything he did for me he is the man who saved my life. Then in 2004 I had and ICD put in, and luckily in the 14 years I've had it, nothing has ever happened. In 2016 I was upgraded to an AICD."

Thanks for sharing this story.

Mark F.   *Derby, KS*   (#102)

Mark has been in our CHF world for 4 months.

The main symptoms he experiences are explained as:

"Sudden weight gain, Edema , pain and Shortness of Breath"

CHF has impacted his quality of life described like this:

"Being able to work"

Mark is being treated with medications:

"Furosemide, Metoprolol and Lisinopril."

He is experiencing Depression/ Anxiety described like this:

"No energy...scared."

He says the worst thing about CHF is:

"Scared about leaving my wife a widow."

This is the story she wanted to share:

"My journey has just started. I go between being angry and denial."

Thanks for sharing this story.

Teresa S.   Daviston, AL   (#103)

Teresa has been in our CHF world for 8 years.

The main symptoms she experiences are explained as:

"Sudden weight gain and Shortness of Breath"

CHF has impacted her quality of life described like this:

"I don't have the energy I used to have. My EF is normal, but my quality of life has decreased due to lack of energy and inability to do the things I used to do"

Teresa is being treated with medications:

"Carvedilol, Enalapril and Lasix."

She is experiencing Depression/ Anxiety described like this:

"Depression, Anxiety caused me to lose my job, affects my family and their ability to spend a lot of time with me"

She says the worst thing about CHF is:

"No energy."

This is the story she wanted to share:

"Diagnosed at 47- it took me 3 dr visits to 3 different clinics to be diagnosed. My EF was 27 when I was diagnosed and I was out of work for 6 months. My EF is 55 now but I feel worse than when I was diagnosed."

Thanks for sharing this story.

Laurie L.   *New Sharon, ME*   (#104)

Laurie has been in our CHF world for 1 1/2 years.

The main symptoms she experiences are explained as:

"Sudden weight gain, Memory Loss, Dizziness, Pain and Shortness of Breath."

CHF has impacted her quality of life described like this:

"I can no longer do the things I used to. I'm tired, and have a hard time breathing. My anxiety and depression levels are through the roof"

Laurie is being treated with medications:

"Carvedilol and also a water pill."

She is experiencing Depression/ Anxiety described like this:

"Yes. I constantly worry about dying, I do not drive much anymore due to the fact that I am scared that my heart will give out and I will hurt or kill someone."

She says the worst thing about CHF is:

"All of it. There is nothing good about CHF."

This is the story she wanted to share:

"I went to the ER with Pneumonia, I totally bottomed out with Sepsis. I was transferred to another hospital better equipped to handle me. I was in a coma like state for a week. When I woke up I found out I had CHF and my EF is 10% and also had diabetes. I spent another week in the hospital. Three months after being discharged from the hospital I had a pacemaker/defibrillator combo implanted. All of this was in June of 2017. So here I am praying every night before bed that I wake up in the morning."

Thanks for sharing this story.

Carrie   *Little Egg Harbor, NJ (#105)*

Carrie has been in our CHF world for 4 years.

The main symptoms she experiences are explained as:

"Edema and Shortness of Breath."

CHF has impacted her quality of life described like this:

"My quality of life suffers as I can no longer do the things I used to do. The Edema, shortness of breath limit my activities as well as my food choices. Going out to eat and drink with friends and family is limited now as I feel so bad afterwards, I don't want to go anymore. Also, the meds and the lack of exercise for the first year after diagnosis caused me to gain 25 lbs so the extra weight not only slows me down but is embarrassing."

Carrie is being treated with medications:

"Blood pressure meds such as Entresto and Coreg even though I have always had low blood pressure. I was on a cholesterol pill - Lipitor - even though I have always had good cholesterol numbers. These pills are the "cocktail of pills" given for CHF. The Lipitor caused my liver to become inflamed so I was taken off of that. It was also causing my joints to ache so I was happy to be taken off of it. Since I still don't have a cholesterol issue, my doctor doesn't feel the need to replace it. I am also on Lasix and Potassium pill daily."

She is experiencing Depression/ Anxiety described like this:

"The first 18 months I suffered from depression but I have overcome that and learned to accept and live with the disease the best I can."

She says the worst thing about CHF is:

"The increase in Edema which causes the shortness of breath which causes the inability to get things done like I used to be able to do. A small variation in what I eat can cause the Edema. I also am tired a lot of the time and not knowing when I am going to feel good or have a bad day. If I have a good day and overdo it, I suffer for a day or two after."

This is the story she wanted to share:

"In March of 2014, I was visiting my sister in Arizona. My second night there I went to bed and when I laid down, I couldn't catch my breath. I have always suffered from Asthma, so thought I was having an Asthma attack. If I sat back up, I could breathe again, not well but definitely better, but when I would lay down again, I could not breathe at all. I ended up staying up all night as I wasn't able to lay down. In the morning when everyone woke up, I told them about it and we discussed that she had given me new feather pillows that night and thought maybe I was allergic to them. My ankles were swollen also but we passed that off as they were like that from the airplane ride. I spent the entire trip there thinking I was having a bad time with my Asthma and just used my inhalers and did breathing treatments. After returning home to NJ, I still had problems breathing but it was spring and I was allergic to the pine pollen and thought that was the cause. In June of 2014, I traveled again and when my husband and I stopped at a hotel to stay, the same thing happened to me as did in AZ. When I laid down, I could not catch my breath. I ended up sitting up all night reading and we thought maybe they also had feather pillows. On the drive home I was able to recline my seat a bit and get some

sleep. My breathing didn't really get better but I could prop myself up on some pillows and get some sleep for the next few nights. We got home on a Monday and I was going to start dieting as my son was getting married in 1 month in Costa Rica. I had spent a year planning for this trip with 50 or our family and friends and wanted to lose a few pounds before the big day. I wasn't able to exercise as I was having so much trouble breathing so I started taking Prednisone on Wednesday. This is usually the miracle drug for Asthma patients but by Thursday night it had done nothing for me. On Friday morning my ankles and feet were swollen so much and when I weighed myself I saw that I had gained 14 pounds since Monday. I decided I couldn't go to Costa Rica like this so I made an appointment to see my doctor that afternoon as I knew it wasn't my Asthma. The minute my doctor saw me he suggested they call an ambulance and take me to the ER. I declined the ambulance and told them I would drive myself. He suggested I not drive so I called my husband at work to pick me up and take me in. At the ER, they immediately did a chest x-ray and could see my enlarged heart. They did an EKG and noticed I was in AFIB. They did an Echocardiogram and my EF was 25%. I was given IV Lasix to remove the fluid and given an ultrasound on my legs to see if I had any blood clots which I did not have. The ER doctor told my husband that I was very sick and she hoped I responded to treatment, but if I didn't, she would recommend he contact hospice. I spent 3 days at that hospital. I was then taken by ambulance to a heart and lung hospital for a heart catheterization. This test showed my arteries were clear. I was diagnosed with Non-Ischemic Dilated Cardiomyopathy, Left Bundle Branch Block, and Congestive Heart Failure. They told me at the time I would need a CRT-D implanted to pace my heart and give me a defibrillator to protect me from Sudden Cardiac Death. After 6 days in the hospital I was sent home on many meds - Coreg, Lisinopril, Lipitor, Lasix and Potassium as well as oxygen. I was told not to do anything strenuous or stressful. Insurance required me to be on the meds for 3 months to see if my EF improved before they would approve the CRT-D implant. I was scheduled to see a cardiologist every month, a pulmonary doctor every month and also an Electrophysiologist for the CRT-D. As I learned more about CHF I tried to figure out when my problems started and what symptoms I missed. I have no family history of heart problems. I realized that for the past couple of years I would often break out in a massive sweat on little exertion or even if I was feeling a bit nervous. I still don't know why that happened but it doesn't happen like it did so I am convinced it is due to the heart problems. For several months prior to diagnosis, I had been very tired and fatigued and I would take 3-4 naps a day. I passed it off as getting older and lazy although now I know that is due to the heart failure. The doctors all said the CHF must have been caused by a virus but to this day I don't know when that could have happened or how long I have had CHF as whenever I was short of breath, I blamed it on my asthma. Since I never liked going to the doctor, I would treat myself for my "asthma attacks". In December of 2014, the CRT-D was implanted. My life began to improve after this as I was able to walk a little more and had a little more stamina. Within 6 months my EF had improved to 35%. In July 2015, I was taken off Lisinopril and put on Entresto. I immediately felt better on Entresto. I didn't retain as much fluid which improved my shortness of breath. In July of 2017, my EF improved to 45%. This is where I stand today. My life isn't great and I will never be able to do what I used to do, but I am a lot better than I was 4 years ago and I am grateful for that.."

Thanks for sharing this story.

Annette F.   *Storvreta, Uppsala, Sweden (#106)*

Annette has been in our CHF world for 1 year.

The main symptoms she experiences are explained as:

"Memory Loss, Shortness of Breath and Tiredness."

CHF has impacted her quality of life described like this:

"Limited to how much I can do in everyday life, for example work, exercise, being with friends, etc"

Annette is being treated with medications:

"Bisoprolol, Spironolactone and Losartan."

She does not experience Depression/ Anxiety but described it like this:

"No, I have to live my life even though I'm ill. It's important for me to stay positive, but that doesn't mean that I'm not sad about my diagnosis."

She says the worst thing about CHF is:

"Not knowing why I got it. Not knowing how long I will live or how long it will take for me to get worse."

This is the story she wanted to share:

"Before I was diagnosed I could hardly walk, but the problem was that I looked too healthy. I had lost weight and I was extremely tired, but was sent home from the doctors. There is nothing wrong with you, was the answer I got when I seeked help. I had pneumonia 6 months before and the problem was that I felt that I was not getting any better. I felt worse and very tired, and I could hear a bubbling noise from my chest. My doctor told me I had a cold. It wasn't until I went to the ER a month later that I was diagnosed with Idiopathic HF. The problem is that I'm too healthy to have this problem. No high bloodpressure, no other illnesses like thyroid problems, I don't drink and I don't smoke, I'm not overweight and I exercise. So... life is not fair, but here I am with this horrible illness. But I'm staying positive and I enjoy life everyday. I look after myself with healthy food (vegan) and I exercise everyday. I have a loving family and friends that support me. I'm lucky in so many ways and I will never stop fighting my illness."

Thanks for sharing this story.

Dion M.   Brisbane, Queensland, Australia (#107)

Dion has been in our CHF world for 4 years.

The main symptoms he experiences are explained as:

"Sudden Weight gain, Edema and Shortness of Breath."

CHF has impacted his quality of life described like this:

"It's shortened my life and taken my quality of life. I can no longer work so have no source of income and can't keep up with my grandson."

Dion is being treated with medications:

"Blood pressure, anticoagulant, beta blockers, fluid retention stopper. The usual types I guess.."

He is experiencing Depression/ Anxiety described like this:

"Very much so. My life as I knew it has gone and I'll never get it back. My new life is bearly a life at all."

He says the worst thing about CHF is:

"Loosing the life you had."

This is the story he wanted to share:

"My wife and I had plans of us both working until retirement and then retiring to a quiet country town. Suddenly that future was lost. Now only my wife can work and we struggle to make ends meet. We no longer expected to be financially secure come retirement age and I don't even expect to reach retirement age. This is not what I wanted for my lovely wife."

Thanks for sharing this story.

Christy   *Los Alamos, NM*   (#108)

Christy has been in our CHF world for 8 years.

The main symptom she experiences are explained as:

> *"Edema, Memory Loss, Dizziness, Shortness of Breath and Depression/Anxiety."*

CHF has impacted her quality of life described like this:

> *"Lost job, insurance, confidence, ability to garden, clean house, etc. Stopped yoga and daily walks in woods near home, which kept me feeling joyous. More."*

Christy is being treated with medications:

> *"Six heart-specific meds; one antidepressant (SNRI)."*

She is experiencing Depression/ Anxiety described like this:

> *"Of course! Affects and colors everything I contemplate. Diminished capacities in everthing!."*

She says the worst thing about CHF is:

"Worries--am I getting worse, will a sudden shock cause a MI, will I be a vegetable from a stroke, can I remain self-sufficient?."

This is the story she wanted to share:

"There isn't room enough and I'm too tired."

Thanks for sharing this information.

Clay L.   *Reno, NV*   (#109)

Clay has been in our CHF world for just 8 months.

The main symptoms he experiences are explained as:

"Dizziness, Shortness of Breath and Lack of Energy."

CHF has impacted his quality of life described like this:

"Can no longer work and depression."

Clay is being treated with medications:

"Baby aspirin, Amiodarone, Atorvastatin, Carvedilol, Clopidogrel, Losartan and Spironolactone."

He is experiencing Depression/ Anxiety described like this:

"Yes, Depression. I have no desire to go anywhere or do anything thing."

He says the worst thing about CHF is:

"Weakness and always dizzy."

This is the story he wanted to share:

"I had my first heart attack in February. They put two stents in and prescribed meds one being Brilanta. Was doing ok but being new to taking meds I missed a few doses. A few months later, I passed out at work and went to the ER. After all the tests I was told that my stents had closed up and that a section of my heart was dead. My EF was 10-15% and was told I might need bypass surgery. They were able to get my artery to open back up and they sent me home with a life vest. About a month later, I passed out and had another heart attack. After being rushed to the ER I was given a AICD implant and a new regiment of meds that I now follow to the letter. My EF is up to 30-35%. I am still dizzy and light headed and cannot work do to the fact I can't stand more than a few minutes every day. They are trying to adjust my meds to help with this. But it seems to be a up hill battle. So I wait."

Thanks for sharing this story.

Vivian M.   Jefferson City, MO   (#110)

Vivian has been in our CHF world for 4 years.

The main symptom she experiences are explained as:

"Edema."

CHF has impacted her quality of life described like this:

"I've had to slow down, can't do things I used to do."

Vivian is being treated with medications:

"Losartan, Coreg and Furosemide."

She is experiencing Depression/ Anxiety described like this:

"Yes, sleep issues, fear and anxiety."

She says the worst thing about CHF is:

"Knowing it is chronic and will probably exacerbate at some point."

This is the story she wanted to share:

"I had come home from a stressful business trip and suddenly had trouble breathing. Went to ER and was diagnosed with Cardiomyopathy. Possibly broken heart syndrome, although my EF has not improved. I have had several episodes since of flash pulmonary Edema. Tried several medications and have a good cardiologist. I also went to counseling for depression."

Thanks for sharing this story.

Melinda   McGaheysville, VA   (#111)

Melinda has been in our CHF world for 2 years.

The main symptoms she experiences are explained as:

"Sudden weight gain, Edema, Memory Loss, Dizziness, Pain and Shortness of Breath."

CHF has impacted her quality of life described like this:

"I can't do my daily chores. I have a hard time getting dressed. And my shopping is strictly online or family does it."

Melinda is being treated with medications:

"Imdur, Renexa, Plavix, asprin, nitroglycerin, beta blockers they seem to change often, Lasix and Crestor."

She is experiencing Depression/ Anxiety described like this:

"I have a fear of going to sleep so I take Xanax."

She says the worst thing about CHF is:

"Not being able to do for my kids."

This is the story she wanted to share:

"It started when I was 36 as a pain in my rib. They treated me for Gastroparesis and a pinched nerve. I had over 100 visits to the ER was even red flagged for opioids. The EKG stress test and Echo always showed normal so I was sent home. A year later they did a Cath and found five blockages I had a quadruple bypass CABG and four months later went through the same only this time even the blood work showed normal. I fought for four months before they did another Cath and found the bypass failed leaving the two harvested arteries they put four stents in and that helped but the angina stayed after 12 heart caths two hospitals and six doctors they decided there was nothing invasive that can be done for the diagnosis of micro vascular disease and systolic and diastolic along with CAD and CVD my diabetes are uncontrollable even with IV insulin and now I have NAFL the fluid stays in my belly and hands so makes moving hard"

Thanks for sharing this story.

Linda R.   *Dedham, MA*   (#112)

Linda has been in our CHF world for just 1 year.

The main symptom she experiences are explained as:

"Sudden weight gain."

CHF has impacted her quality of life described like this:

"At first I was afraid to do anything but after attending cardiac rehab I started doing more and joining this group. I learned people have lived years with CHF giving me hope. I've also followed a Loso diet which again this group has done a lot to educate me about!!"

Linda is being treated with medications:

"Diuretic and long acting nitro."

She is experiencing Depression/ Anxiety described like this:

"I do meditation daily and keep my relationships close!"

She says the worst thing about CHF is:

"Constantly watching what I eat and checking my weight.."

This is the story she wanted to share:

"I unexpectedly had angina one evening, ended up in the ER and after some test ended up having open heart with double bypass. During my 3 month of recovery, I had angina again! I had a catherization and they discovered my graft was blocking because it was stitched too tight! During the catherization they did a balloon angioplasty to open the graph. That unfortunately only lasted less than a month and back in I went and had another catherization with a stent placed in the graph. That was only 3 months ago and I'm still recovering. My CHF episode happened 2 months ago and thus a loso diet."

Thanks for sharing this story.

Pauline H. Luton, Bedfordshire, UK   (#113)

Pauline has been in our CHF world for 4 years.

The main symptoms she experiences are explained as:

"Sudden weight gain, Edema, Pain and Shortness of Breath."

CHF has impacted her quality of life described like this:

"Complete 180. Gave up work. Feel isolated and useless have time. Sick of feeling sick"

Pauline is being treated with medications:

"Spironolactone, Atorvastatin, Bisoporolol, Clopidogrel and aspirin."

She is experiencing Depression/ Anxiety described like this:

"Both. Low mood and tearful all the time. Panic attacks fear of leaving my home."

She says the worst thing about CHF is:

"Breathless and sweating on minimal effort. Scared all time gonna die. No one understands my feelings."

This is the story she wanted to share:

"Rheumatoid Arthritis & Fibromyalgia and use of steroids caused damage to my heart. Had first September 4 2015, second September 5, 2017 followed by cardiac arrest with down time of 14mins on September 6, 2017. Routine follow up show progressive reduction in heart function, 57% now 37%. Waiting to on more test to see if I'm a candidate for a defibrillator. Life is currently living in limbo, life is constant pain and fear."

Thanks for sharing this story.

Charlene A.   Fulton, MO   (#114)

Charlene has been in our CHF world since diagnosed Feb. 26, 2018.

The main symptoms she experiences are explained as:

"Dizziness and Shortness of Breath."

CHF has impacted her quality of life described like this:

"It has had a huge impact on my life, I had to change my eating, start counting sodium, stop drinking caffeine, and stop smoking. (I smoked for 30+ years). I can not do alot of things that I took for granted, like slow jogging and or long walks with my dog. I can't handle the heat anymore, so if the temperature and humidity is over a certain number, I can't be outside or I start breathing like I have a elephant sitting on my chest. So all the outdoor activities I used to do outside, I can no longer do. The only good impact it has on my life is I stopped smoking."

Charlene is being treated with medications:

"Lasix, Carvedilol, Spironolactone, Lisinopril. I was put on 3 more due to my AFIB yesterday, but dont know what they are yet because I am in the hospital."

She is experiencing Depression/ Anxiety described like this:

"I had depression and anxiety before I was diagnosed with CHF. But sometimes my depression and anxiety is worse due to CHF. It effects me as in, alot of times I just sit and obsess that I'm going to die, or asked what did I do to deserve this, why me, then I obsess on that it's because of my past and all the partying I did. It's just an emotional roller coaster ride."

She says the worst thing about CHF is:

"I am an EXTREMELY independent person, so the worst thing about having CHF is not being able to do some of the things I used to do, I hate asking people to help me."

This is the story she wanted to share:

"I found out I had CHF when I kept waking up in the middle of the night gasping for breath, but I let it go on for a week because the last thought on my mind was it had something to do with my heart. I was devastated when I was told I had CHF and my EF was 10%. I literally thought I was going to die in days. All I could do for days and days was to cry. The doctor didnt know what caused my CHF which made things worse for me. I was a ex meth addict (been clean for 13 years) and I kept obsessing on that was why I had CHF, and I beat myself up over that. My husband was in prison, (he became addicted to pain pills when he broke his back and did some stupid stuff) so of course I obsessed on what was going to happen to my 12 year old son, who is my life. I wasn't ready to die. I was scared to die, but now I know I was scared of what I would miss out on if I died. I worried how my son would grow up because I have always been determined that my son had a better life than me. Finally my husband came home, my work (work at a deaf school 19 years) supported me, but the biggest support came from the Congestive Heart Failure group, I joined on Facebook. This group was absolutely amazing. So many strangers making *me feel better with prayers and encouraging words and they knew how I felt and where I was coming from. Although I have never meet these strangers, they are now my CHF family. Anytime I am curious or have a question or just boost my spirits up I can 100% depend on my CHF family. In May 2018, I got my 2nd echo, (after wearing a miserable life vest for 3 months) my EF went to 25%. Of course, that's an improvement and I should have been happy but I wasnt. I had high hopes and faith that my EF would be higher because I stopped smoking, changed my eating, etc. Then the same day the doctor tells me that I need a ICD implant and scheduled the surgery for like 5 days later. I was once again devastated. On June 6, 2018, I had surgery and got my implant. I now of course know it was a good thing and no more life vest! Thank God! So slowly but surely I started accepting my CHF, (most days). I had so many life changes happen to me in 4 months, it was hard on my mind and body. Now 6 months after being diagnosed with CHF, I am sitting in the hospital because I have also been diagnosed with AFIB. For the 3rd time in 6 months I am yet devastated again, but this time it feels worse. I am 10 times more scared of having AFIB. I try to wrap my mind around it but it's hard. I've asked my CHF family a few questions about AFIB, but I havent talked about being diagnosed with it yet. I feel like I don't have the energy, but yet I'm sitting here typing this. Strange- I know.."*

Thanks for sharing this story.

Linda P.   *Lancaster, PA*   *(#115)*

Linda has been in our CHF world for just 6 months.

The main symptoms she experiences are explained as:

"Edema, Dizziness and Shortness of Breath."

CHF has impacted her quality of life described like this:

"Greatly impacted. I swell so bad I can't walk"

Linda is being treated with medications:

"Tursomide."

She is experiencing Depression/ Anxiety described like this:

"Yes, shortness of breath and can't sleep."

She says the worst thing about CHF is:

"Unknowns."

This is the story she wanted to share:

"My journey has just begun but I am scared, very scared. Is this the end of my life?"

Thanks for sharing this story.

Nettie O.   *Cork, Cork, Ireland*   *(#116)*

Nettie has been in our CHF world for 1 year.

The main symptoms she experiences are explained as:

"Edema, Memory Loss, Diziness, Fatique and Exercise Intolerance."

CHF has impacted her quality of life described like this:

"I've had to retire early and I have very poor quality of life right now. I'm hoping that will change soon though."

Nettie is being treated with medications:

"Beta blocker and loop diuretic."

She is experiencing Depression/ Anxiety described like this:

"It's only 3 months since diagnosis and it has only hit me this week."

She says the worst thing about CHF is:

"Having NO energy and no stamina and also that loved ones don't understand.."

This is the story she wanted to share:

"Being a nurse I knew I had heart failure. But I did not seek medical attention because I just wanted the whole thing to disappear. I was in denial and also I was busy looking after a very ill teenager, so my own health always was of least importance. But now I've been diagnosed 3 months. I was put on medication and sent on my merry way with no real education or advice. I'm having all my tests repeated next week and then follow up shortly after. As I approached this 3 month mark with no support (not even a leaflet), I realize that I actually feel worse than when I started on my meds. I have no energy, and have difficulty breathing most of the time. Mostly, I am housebound. I was not warned how bad the meds would make me feel initially. I know I am early in this journey so far so do not have too much to share. But, I can say that it has been a very lonely journey so far. As I realize that I am no better off after 3 months of meds, the reality of heart failure has just hit me. I am sad, angry and very scared. My life is on hold until I have more answers and this is no way to exist. My youngest child is only 18."

Thanks for sharing this story.

Amanda G.   Hickory, NC   (#117)

Amanda has been in our CHF world for 1 year.

The main symptoms she experiences are explained as:

"Memory Loss, Dizziness and Shortness of Breath."

CHF has impacted her quality of life described like this:

"CHF has had a huge impact on my life. Constant medicine, exhaustion, shortness of breath, lack of sleep, hospital visits, insane amount of doctor appointments, sweating, not being able to tolerate the heat anymore and not being able to be the parent I once was."

Amanda is being treated with medications:

"Metoprolol, Spironolactone, Entresto and aspirin."

She is experiencing Depression/ Anxiety described like this:

"I have had pretty bad depression since I found out I had CHF. Not knowing what the future holds is scary, and the chance that I could leave my kids is really depressing..."

She says the worst thing about CHF is:

"The symptoms. Mainly lack of energy and shortness of breath. Can't do what I want to anymore.."

This is the story she wanted to share:

"It will be a year in January since I found out I had CHF. I tried to go to sleep one night and when I laid down I couldn't breathe. I felt like I was hyperventilating. I'm 29 and a single mother of a 5 and 6 year old. Not wanting to wake the kids, I decided to wait till the morning to go to the doctor. When I went to the doctor my blood pressure and heart rate was so high they immediately sent me to the ER. They ran a lot of tests and found out my lungs were full of fluid. They then admitted me to the ICU. After getting a bit of fluid out of my lungs they sent me for a stress test. I thought I was going home, but the cardio team came in and told me that my stress test came back not good. My EF was 25% and I had Congestive Heart Failure. I didn't even know what it meant at the time, and I was scared to death. The doctor explained it as my heart was that of a 70 to 80 year old. I was put on medicine and my strict low sodium diet. Finally after a week, I was allowed to go home. It became a new life though. I no longer can do the things I used to. I am tired all the time, get out of breath really quick, qnd constantly sweat. I can't handle the heat, and I definitely can't go outside and play with my kids like I used to. Which is really hard being a single mother. It's still new to me, but has caused a lot more problems than just with my heart. My kidneys are failing also, and they might have to take my pancreas out. We don't know what the future holds, but I have faith everything will work out. Just a big lifestyle change.."

Thanks for sharing this story.

Nikki W.   *Centerton, AR*   *(#118)*

Nikki has been in our CHF world for 3 years.

The main symptoms she experiences are explained as:

"Edema, Dizziness and Shortness of Breath."

CHF has impacted her quality of life described like this:

"My quality of life was already diminished due to my CSF leak otherwise known as Cerebrospinal fluid (CSF) fluid leak or Spontaneous Cerebral Hypotension which caused my CHF. It is harder to breathe, walk with out being tired. You have to watch your fluid intake and sodium which is needed for the spinal leak. Heat plays a toll on you. Doctors dont want to treat you for other problems because of the heart problems."

Nikki is being treated with medications:

"Tourisimide, Entresto, Carvedilol and Corlanor."

She is experiencing Depression/ Anxiety described like this:

"Anxiety. I worry about not waking up in the morning."

She says the worst thing about CHF is:

"Not being able to breathe."

This is the story she wanted to share:

"My face swelled up and I couldnt breathe one night. My doctor ordered a Echocardiogram and the hospital wouldn't let me leave until a cardiologist saw me. My EF was 15% and I have had numerous heart caths. One with an impeler for a stent to be placed which resulted in a helicopter ride to another hospital and 2 severe blood loss episodes. I have had a Cardiomem implanted to help keep track of my fluid retention also. My heart failure is unique because the doctors can not figure out how to give me the correct meds without causing more problems with my CSF leak. The meds and my CSF leak don't go together."

Thanks for sharing this story.

Leigh Ann B.   *Gray, LA*   (#119)

Leigh has been in our CHF world as explained:

"I got my diagnosis in Feb. 2018, but I'm pretty sure I have had CHF for a couple of years."

The main symptoms she experiences are explained as:

"Edema and Shortness of Breath."

CHF has impacted her quality of life described like this:

"I have made some dietary changes and quit smoking. Medications and I am feeling almost normal. A little tired sometimes."

Leigh is being treated with medications:

"Coreg, Lasix, Spironolactone and Lisinipril."

She is experiencing Depression/ Anxiety described like this:

"Depression at first. But I got over it."

She says the worst thing about CHF is:

_____

"Giving up salty foods."

_____

This is the story she wanted to share:

_____

"After months of a cough that would not go away, and swelling in my lower legs, which my Dr said was nothing. I went to the ER with what I thought was Bronchitis, I was admitted and diagnosed with CHF."

_____

Thanks for sharing this story.

LaVonda S.   *Jacksonville, FL (#120)*

LaVonda has been in our CHF world for 2 years.

The main symptoms she experiences are explained as:

"Sudden Weight Gain, Edema, Memory Loss and Shortness of Breath."

CHF has impacted her quality of life described like this:

"Initially, I was scared to close my eyes at night, so I was very fearful, overwhelmed, and anxious about my new norm. I definitely can't do as much as I used to without stopping numerous times and it's a little lonely."

LaVonda is being treated with medications:

"Diuretics, Blood Pressure and Heart Failure Meds."

She is experiencing Depression/ Anxiety described like this:

"It gets frustrating because people look at you and just assume that nothing is really wrong because it can't be seen or that you are just being lazy. Often times, people don't understand your limitations and fatigue. Depression creeps in from time to time, but every new day brings an opportunity to make life changes for the improvement of yourself."

She says the worst thing about CHF is:

"For me personally, it was not knowing my limitations for fluid and salt intake. Not knowing landed me in the E.R. from an overload. I didnt know the signs or symptoms that I was in trouble or needed to seek assistance."

This is the story she wanted to share:

"I was 46 when my journey started. I was coughing a lot and found it hard to breathe laying flat to sleep at night, which was unusual for me. Then I started realizing that I couldn't walk from the parking lot to my office building without shortness of breath and sweating profusely. This went on for a week or so, before I realized that I couldn't walk from my desk to the cafe at work without the same symptoms, plus my clothes were getting extremely tight. So I finally got scared enough to get myself evaluated. I was then told that I was experiencing Congestive Heart Failure and need to get rid of the extra fluid. From there, I started going to the CHF clinic where I learned more about my condition such as the signs and symptoms to look out for, my intake restrictions, diet and nutrition tips, and what exercises I could do safely. I feel more confident 2 yrs later and understand my limitations and why. I also have a new found love for cooking and exploring new healthy food options. Last but not least, I have found a lot of great people just like me in my support groups, so now I am not lonely anymore."

Thanks for sharing this story.

Wendi T.   Batavia, IL   (#121)

Wendi has been in our CHF world for 1 1/2 years.

The main symptoms she experiences are explained as:

"Edema, Memory Loss, Dizziness, Shortness of Breath and Gout."

CHF has impacted her quality of life described like this:

"Causes a lot of depression and anxiety. Can't do as much as I use to. Not being able to work."

Wendi is being treated with medications:

"Lopressor and Losartan."

She is experiencing Depression/ Anxiety described like this:

"Yes, panic attacks, over sensitive and emotional. Makes me not want to socialize like a use to and be a loner."

She says the worst thing about CHF is:

"The unknown."

This is the story she wanted to share:

"I randomly found out I had CHF. I had broken my foot and was sedentary for over a year. I then sprained my other ankle and the swelling never went away. I became breathless and fatigued. Went to ER and they did a Probnp blood test and it came back high. I was release with an order for an Echo. A week later I get the Echo and I'm called the next day and told to get into my doctor as soon as possible. My EF was only 20%. I was devastated, my dad had just died two months before this and my first thought was now I'm going to die. Over the next year I worked my butt off doing everything the doctors told me to do and I'm happy to report that as of this last week my EF is now 42%."

Thanks for sharing this story.

Carole R.   *Pelham, NH*   (#122)

Carole has been in our CHF world for 3 years.

The main symptoms she experiences are explained as:

"Sudden Weight Gain, and Shortness of Breath."

CHF has impacted her quality of life described like this:

"It has been very difficult, some days are good and some aren't. I try to watch my sodium intake, but that also such a burden. I also have stage four COPD so you could say I'm constantly out of breath. But I do the best I can, I get up, get dressed and make sure I get at least one task done in my house everyday."

Carole is being treated with medications:

"Bumex and Metoprolol."

She is experiencing Depression/ Anxiety described like this:

"Absolutely, I cry a lot I have tried so many medications but nothing seems to work. I do have a beautiful granddaughter age two and when she's around I can't stop smiling."

She says the worst thing about CHF is:

"For me it's the exhaustion. I feel after sleeping ten hours, then I need a nap three hours later."

This is the story she wanted to share:

"I had open heart surgery three years ago, 2015. I never even knew I had CHF until three years later. I had an attack and was in the hospital for one week. The worst thing about the disease is you can't see it. If my leg was broken and in a cast people are right there to help you up, etc.. But nobody gets it with CHF! It does cause you to gain weight so that constantly bothers me, and of course people can't help but say"oh you've gained a few pounds as if I didn't know. I truly believe my husband and daughter understand but not friends, I've even lost friends because I can't do what I use to , they don't understand so I'm never invited. That in itself is so painful to me it makes me feel like my life as I knew it is over. I have a portable oxygen but who wants to use that going out? Not me I'll stay home. You know they have the CHF groups and sometimes it cheers me up other times not so much. You get people that say oh, ' I have stage one COPD (mild) and CHF and I run three miles four times a week.' Now I can honestly tell you nobody in this group gives a shit. Your just here to brag and make everyone else feel bad about themselves. Especially when it's an effort to climb up the stairs. I don't know if I'm just jealous or I hate them for being able to run. Then I get mean (in my mind) and I say to myself "wait until they get to stages 3-4 then let's hear you brag). But you know what, prior to 2015 I have had a good life, a wonderful husband for forty three years, a beautiful daughter and granddaughter. I lived through the drug era mostly because I didn't participate. Lived longer than alot of my friends, have a beautiful home so I'm grateful I'm still here. I do what I'm told for the most part, I can't control the future I just thank God each morning when I wake up. What's most important is that doctors definitely need to be more honest with there patients and explain things in detail. And these doctors that give patients the number of years they may have left. What the hell so you sit at home crying away the day, weeks, months,

years, just waiting. Their not God, none of us have an expiration date stamped on the bottom of our feet, each one of us is different and we all need to remember that. May God Bless us all. ❤✉ *"*

Thanks for sharing this story.

Joni M.   Houston, TX   (#123)

Joni has been in our CHF world for 2 years.

The main symptoms she experiences are explained as:

"Sudden Weight gain, Edema and Shortness of Breath."

CHF has impacted her quality of life described like this:

"Just cannot do the things I used to, no stamina anymore."

Joni is being treated with medications:

"Lasix, Coreg and Potassium."

She is <u>not</u> experiencing Depression/ Anxiety.

She says the worst thing about CHF is:

"Lack of stamina and therefore loss of some quality of life."

This is the story she wanted to share:

"I began having shortness of breath to the point where I couldn't sleep laying down anymore, also I felt like I had swallowed a bowling ball. I went to my GP and she tested me for all kinds of things, didn't find anything. I then went to a pulmonologist and he took one look at my swollen legs and said I had CHF. I had a couple of tests and that was confirmed. Once I got onto a Coreg and Lasix regimen. I lost nearly 60 pounds of water weight and have had it under control for over a year now."

Thanks for sharing this story.

Teresa D.   Gainesville, FL   (#124)

Teresa has been in our CHF world for 2 years.

The main symptoms she experiences are explained as:

"Sudden weight gain and Dizziness."

CHF has impacted her quality of life described like this:

"I don't go out like I used to. It's hard to go out to eat with people. I don't date because I don't think someone would want a sick person."

Teresa is being treated with medications:

"Lisinopril, Metoprolol, Spironolactone and Lasix."

She is experiencing Depression/ Anxiety described like this:

"Not too much. I try to stay positive."

She says the worst thing about CHF is:

"I hate feeling like I might die soon."

This is the story she wanted to share:

"I was shocked with my diagnosis. I just thought I had an upper respiratory infection. After my diagnosis, it was really scary researching it on the internet. It seemed like a death sentence. I was lucky to find a Facebook support group that helped with learning healthy low sodium foods and offered me an optimistic outlook on things. I have a pacemaker/ defibrillator now and I feel fortunate to be healthy and doing well. I am still able to work and I enjoy a fairly normal life."

Thanks for sharing this story.

Sam P.   *Ramsgate, Kent, UK*   (#125)

Sam has been in our CHF world for 3 years.

The main symptoms he experiences are explained as:

"Dizziness, Excessive Sweating, but mainly no symptoms now."

CHF has impacted his quality of life described like this:

"Has caused me Great Depression and anxiety living with an uncertain condition. Luckily, I am able to live life almost as before with my stable dilated cardiomyopathy."

Sam is not being treated with medications.

He is experiencing Depression/ Anxiety described like this:

"Yes, this diagnosis is a constant burden to me and worries me a lot. I want to live a long time and see my children grow up and when you have a heart condition things are so uncertain. I try and focus on the fact that I mainly have no symptoms and my heart is improving."

He says the worst thing about CHF is:

"The uncertainty of the future and people not really understanding the condition."

This is the story he wanted to share:

"I became extremely ill in October 2015 with what seemed like a virus. I went to my doctor with symptoms of shortness of breath and fast heart rate but was not really taken seriously and was sent away with an Asthma inhaler. I preceded to get more and more poorly, couldn't lie down flat, couldn't eat, couldn't sleep and was swelling so eventually had to go to my local accident and emergency department (I almost passed out on the way). I then spent a month in hospital and was diagnosed with dilated cardiomyopathy, heart failure and multiple blood clots on the lungs. At this point I was only 28 years old. I was put on Bumetanide, Furosemide, Spironolactone, Ivabradine, Bisoprolol, Ramipril and Riveroxaban. My EF was 10-14% at this time. Also while in hospital they gave me too many blood thinners which caused me to have a gastrointestinal bleed so I ended up in ICU and needed a blood transfusion. Then I developed Sepsis which almost killed me. I very nearly died from this whole experience and being separated from my loved ones was the hardest thing. After a month, I was discharged and spent the next few months determined to feel better so began walking in moderation and trying to live normally, as best I could. Swelling was no longer and issue so I was allowed to discontinue my water pills. Since then I have slowly discontinued my other medications and feel well now. My EF has risen to 45% and my heart is shrinking. I really feel the same as always now which is a relief and feel incredibly lucky for the turn of events. I do still excessively sweat though which I feel must be related to my condition. I am 31 years old now and hope to live a long life with my family. Unfortunately, in my case the side effects of the medications were too much (constant stomach issues, flu like illness, body aches, severe rashes) so I have chosen to take a natural path (taking multiple supplements, eating healthily and walking 3 miles a day) and that seems to be working well for me. I feel privileged to essentially be A-symptomatic. Still, this diagnosis always hangs over me and causes me severe depression at times.."

Thanks for sharing this story.

Michael N.   *Richland, MS*   (#126)

Michael has been in our CHF world for just 1 year.

The main symptoms he experiences are explained as:

"Sudden Weight Gain, Edema, Mamory Loss, Pain and Shortness of Breath."

CHF has impacted his quality of life described like this:

"Limits my everyday actions."

Michael is being treated with medications:

"Carvidilol, Elequis and Entresto."

He is experiencing Depression/ Anxiety described like this:

"Both, it's affecting my work performance."

He says the worst thing about CHF is:

"Fear of death."

This is the story he wanted to share:

"Diagnosed in July of 2017 in conjunction with AFIB. Numerous hospital stays, Med trials and errors."

Thanks for sharing this story.

Steven H.   Portland, OR   (E01)

Steven has been in our CHF world for only 1 year.

The main symptoms he experiences are explained as:

"SOB, memory loss, puffy legs and head rushes."

CHF has impacted his quality of life described like this:

"It has had a tremendous impact on my life, I work 40 hours a week in a US Army Corps of Engineers warehouse, I do moderate to heavy physical work. I am unable to work at my previous level, things that were simple for me are now a lot harder and more tiring. By Fridays I am wiped out, earlier if I had a very taxing week. I lost my CDL to drive bus for my church, I have driven for 14 years, and had my CDL for 30+ years, that was really hard for me. "

Steven is being treated with medications.

Losartan Potassium, Fluconazole, Fluoxetine HCl, Carvedilol, Amlodipine Besylate, Potassium Chloride, Torsemide, Spironolactone, Atorvastatin Calcium and Aspirin 81 MG

He is experiencing Depression/ Anxiety described like this:

"I have had depression since I was a child, so I can't tell that. I know that I am sadder because of CHF."

He says the worst thing about CHF is:

"Where do I start, I have only had it 1 year, but its already made such a negative impact on my life."

This is the story she wanted to share:

"My journey so far is only a year old. I was diagnosed last September, last April I was taking care my wife after her bilateral knee replacement. I was busy taking care of her and I had completely forgot to take my high blood pressure pills. That said, one night I was giving my wife pain pills, I was about to go back to bed and I just didn't feel good. We called 911, AMR found my Blood pressure was 212 over something. After months of testing I was finally diagnosed in Sept 2017. My sister Lee Jorgensen who is also in the group has CHF. Our Dad had it, which I didn't know or remember until I started seeing some of the pills I take, he took also."

Thanks for sharing this story.

Author's Note

Once again, I want to thank all the group members who submitted their story for this book. The two Facebook groups involved are both private groups. Absolutely __no__ information has been taken from the posts and discussions on those groups. By completing our on-line survey and after reading all the disclaimers in it, they have granted us their permission to use only the survey responses in this book. Some people's names were withheld at their request.

Tom Trimble

CONDITIONS EXPLAINED

This section will help explain the many different conditions and abbreviations mentioned in the Member Responses. We will provide just a very basic description of them, not a medical analysis. Hopefully, the readers can use this as a reference to understand people's entries.

Condition	Abbreviation	Description
Alpha-1		Hereditary lung disease
Atrial Septal Defect	ASD	Congenital heart condition which allows blood flow between the atria
Cardiac Arrest		Abrupt loss of heart function
Chronic Fatigue Syndrome	CFS	A complex disorder characterized by extreme fatigue.
Chronic Obstructive Pulmonary Disease	COPD	Refers to two long-term lung diseases -- chronic bronchitis and emphysema -- that often occur together. COPD makes it hard for you to breathe
Congestive Heart Failure	CHF	Progressive heart disease that affects pumping action of the heart muscle.
Coronary Artery Disease	CAD or CHD	Also called Coronary Heart Disease is a serious condition which results from plaque buildup in the arteries.
Cowden's Syndrome		A disease that can cause benign overgrowths called hamartomas.
Diastolic CHF		Heart failure with preserved left ventricular function.

Dilated Cardiomyopathy		A condition in which the heart becomes enlarged and cannot pump blood effectively.
Edema		A condition characterized by an excess of watery fluid collecting in the cavities or tissues of the body
Fibromuscular Dysplasia	FMD	A condition that causes narrowing (stenosis) and enlargement (aneurysm) of the medium-sized arteries in your body.
Gastric Esophageal Reflux Disease	GERD	Occurs when stomach acid frequently flows back into the tube connecting your mouth and stomach (esophagus)
Hypertrophic Cardiomyopathy	HCOM	Thickening of the heart muscle
Non-Hodgkin's Lymphoma		Cancer that originates in your lymphatic system
Obstructive Sleep Apnea	OSA	Type of sleep apnea which is caused by complete or partial obstructions of the upper airway.
Osteoporosis		Bone weakening disease where fractures can be life-altering
Pleural Effusion		A buildup of fluid in the pleural space, an area between the layers of tissue that line the lungs and the chest cavity.
Premature Ventricular Contraction	PVC	A relatively common event where the heartbeat is initiated by Purkinje fibers in the ventricles rather than by the sinoatrial node, the normal heartbeat initiator.
Pulmonary Hypertension	PH	Pulmonary hypertension is a condition of increased blood pressure within the arteries of the lungs.
Scleroderma		Scleroderma is a group of autoimmune diseases that may result in changes to the skin, blood vessels, muscles, and internal organs.

Supraventricular Tachycardia	SVT	Abnormally fast heart rhythm arising from improper electrical activity in the upper part of the heart
Tetralogy of Fallot	TOF	Tetralogy of Fallot is a type of heart defect present at birth. Symptoms include episodes of bluish color to the skin
Transient Ischemic Attack	TIA	a "mini-stroke" and should be taken very seriously.
Ventricular Fibrillation	VFIB	When the heart quivers instead of pumping due to disorganized electrical activity in the ventricles.
Ventricular Septal Defect	VSD	A defect in the septum between the right and left ventricle.

MEDICATION INFORMATION

This medication information is provided ONLY to help readers to understand the member's posts, where they refer to the medications they take. Please do not use this as a reference for medication decisions. These are only basic references.

Medication	Usage
Adempas	Lowers blood pressure in your lungs
Adriamycin	Chemotherapy medicine
Aldactone	Potassium–sparing diuretic
Allopurinol	Treats gout or kidney stones
Alprazolam	Treat anxiety
Ambien	Sedative for insomnia
Amiodarone	Treats heart rhythm issues
Amitriptyline	Antidepressant
Amlodipine	Treat high blood pressure and angina
ARB (Angiotensin Receptor blocker)	Treats heart failure and prevents kidney failure
Atorvastatin	Statin for cholesterol
Baclofen	Treatment of spastic movements
Bidil	Treats heart failure
Bisoprolol	Beta- Blocker for high blood pressure
Brilinta	Reduces the risk of stroke after a heart attack

Bumex	Diuretic
Bupropion	Help stop smoking
Buspar	Treat anxiety
Buspirone	Treat anxiety
Celebrex	NSAID for inflammation
Cellcept	Prevent organ rejection
Cimetidine	H2 Blocker for stomach acid
Clonazepam	Seizure medication
Clopidogrel (Plavix)	Reduce the risk of stroke
COq10	Antioxidant
Coreg (Carvedilol)	Beta- Blocker for high blood pressure
Corlanor	Treats heart failure
Cosentyx	Treats psoriasis
Crestor	Statin for cholesterol
Cymbalta	Treat depressive disorders
Demadex (Torsemide)	Diuretic
Digitalis	Heart stimulant for rhythm problems
Digoxin	Treat heart failure and slow the heart rate
Dilt-XR	Treat high blood pressure and chest pain
Duloxetine	Help relieve nerve pain, neuropathy
Effient	Prevent blood clots and stroke
Eliquis	Prevent blood clots and stroke
Entresto	Lower blood pressure and treat CHF
Escitalopram	Treats major depression
Famotidine	Treat and prevent ulcers
Gabapentin	Treat seizures and nerve pain
Glimepiride	Treats Diabetes
Glipizide	Treats Diabetes
Humalog	Treat diabetes
Hydralazine	Treats severe hypertension
Hydrodiuril	Thiazide diuretic

Hydroxyzine	Antihistamine for allergies
Irbesartan	Treat high blood pressure and neuropathy
Janumet	Treat Type 2 diabetes
Lansoprazole	Reduce stomach acid
Lasix	Loop diuretic
Levemir	Insulin for diabetes
Levothyroxine	Thyroid medication
Lexapro	Treat anxiety
Liothyronine	Treat underactive Thyroid
Lisinopril	Treat hypertension and CHF
Losartan	Treat high blood pressure and reduce the risk of stroke
Metformin	Treat Type 2 diabetes
Metoprolol	Treat chest pain and high blood pressure
Mexiletine	Antiarrhythmic for heart rhythm
Montelukast	Treat asthma and allergies
Multaq	Treats AFIB
Norpace	Antiarrhythmic for controlling heart rhythms
Norvasc	Relaxes blood vessels and cause your heart to reduce the amount of work required.
Omeprazole	Treat excess stomach acid
Pantoprazole	Treat excess stomach acid
Pepcid	Treat ulcers and stomach acid
Perindopril	Treat high blood pressure and heart failure
Plavix	Prevent blood clots and stroke
Pradaxa	Anticoagulant and help prevent strokes
Pravastatin	Reduce cholesterol and triglycerides
Prednisone	Treat inflammation
Propafenone	Antiarrhythmic for controlling heart rhythms
Prozac	Treat depressive disorders

Ramipril	Treat high blood pressure
Ranexa	Treats angina, chest pain
Ranitidine	Treat stomach acid reflux
Ranitidine	Treat and prevent ulcers
Sertraline	Treat depression and anxiety
Simvastatin	Treat high cholesterol
Sotalol	Serious abnormal heart rhythms
Spironolactone	Treats Edema and preserves potassium
Synthroid	Treat underactive thyroid
Torsemide	Diuretic
Trazadone	Antidepressant
Uloric	Treats gout and lowers blood uric acid
Valsartan	Treats high blood pressure and CHF
Vasotec	Treats high blood pressure and CHF
Veltessa	Used to treat a high level of potassium in your blood.
Venlafaxine	Antidepressant
Warfarin (Coumadin)	Blood Thinner
Wellbutrin	Antidepressant
Xanax	Treat anxiety and panic attacks
Xarelto	Anticoagulant
Zocor	Treat high cholesterol
Zoloft	Treats depression

AUTHORS' THOUGHTS

"In bringing this book to a close, I once again want to thank all the members of the two Congestive Heart Failure Support groups on Facebook. All of them volunteering their stories made up the warm chronical of their Life Journeys presented here. I sincerely hope that this will help people understand how a group like this has worked to survive the progressive monster called CHF. How being told you have CHF is a challenge, not a death sentence. This book presents only their stories and is not intended for medical diagnosis, treatment or even as medical suggestions. Please depend on your medical team for all diagnosis, medication, and treatments. I hope your future Life Journey is as good as possible and as long as possible." Thanks, **Thomas Trimble**

"As you finish our book, I hope that the stories you have read help you understand Congestive Heart Failure and how it affects the lives of real people. Each word is a small expression of the person living with CHF who fights like a warrior to win a battle, which over time will have many casualties. It's the sad reality of CHF. However, as someone living with CHF I know I will fight to the end, as will many of the people in this book as well as the millions of people in the United States and the world diagnosed with this disease.

We want you to remember that Congestive Heart Failure doesn't mean life is over. While many people have the misconception that 'we don't look sick and are just lazy', the truth is we are fighting a battle on the inside of our bodies which rarely manifests itself on the outside of the body. Our limitations are not imaginary. We manage our daily lives so we continue

to function doing as much as we did prior to our diagnosis. And, we have all found support through online groups thru Facebook which allow us to share our failures and successes in dealing with CHF. These groups are the best therapy for many of us! Lastly, thank you for purchasing our book. There are countless untold stories which could be told in hundreds of more books. Take the time to tell your story to your family and friends if you are diagnosed with CHF. If you are a caregiver, use the information in this book to provide top-notch care and share what you have read to help others with CHF. Together, we are all warriors fighting for a victory!"
Thanks, *Jerome Boeck*

"It's amazing that one disease can have so many different combinations of stories, but in the end, all share one common goal. That goal is to live each day to the fullest. It is a silent disease that does not care how young or old you are. This condition can be extra difficult for young people inflicted with it. Many people see young people with CHF as lazy. It is easy to come to that conclusion. Some days you lay in bed all day with no energy. Other days you can get tired and winded walking up a flight of stairs and need to sit for a little while to catch your breath. On good days, that same person can go jog a mile and act like anyone else their age. What I want people to realize is that on bad days, people who exhibit these behaviors, are not lazy. In fact, they are quite the opposite. When just completing everyday tasks make a person with CHF feel like they have just sprinted a mile, that's not lazy. If anything, that person is working harder than you are because the entire day can be a struggle. Want to live a day like a person with CHF? After each task, you do such as getting dressed, taking a shower, getting the mail, vacuuming a room, etc., make yourself do 10 pushups. You will see how quickly doing small tasks takes a toll on your body and why that person is exhausted come dinnertime. This is the daily struggle of someone with CHF. Still think we are lazy? How can you help if you don't *have CHF? Be supportive and there for that person. It's really as simple as that. I can promise we don't want to be this way and would change it if we could. I know I would in a heartbeat. We all live with this each and every day not knowing what tomorrow brings, or even worse if tomorrow will ever come. So, everyone reading this, be happy that your heart is beating and you have breath in your lungs because no matter what is wrong, it could be worse."*

*Thanks, **Christopher Gehrke***

Made in the USA
Coppell, TX
18 March 2024

30243218R00164